Pass the PAX RN!

A Complete NLN PAX RN Study Guide and Practice Test Questions

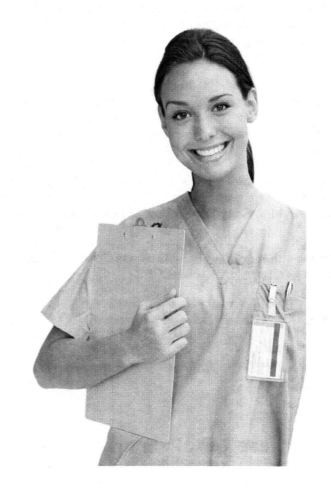

Published by

Complete TEST
Preparation Inc.

ISBN-13: 978-1927358641 (Complete Test Preparation Inc.)
ISBN-10: 1927358647

Version 5.1 February 2014

About Complete Test Preparation Inc.

Complete Test Preparation Inc. has been publishing high quality study materials since 2005. Thousands of students visit our websites every year, and thousands of students, teachers and parents all over the world have purchased our teaching materials, curriculum, study guides and practice tests.

Complete Test Preparation Inc. is committed to providing students with the best study materials and practice tests available on the market. Members of our team combine years of teaching experience, with experienced writers and editors, all with advanced degrees.

Team Members for this publication

Editor: Brian Stocker MA
Contributor: Dr. C. Gregory
Contributor: Dr. G. A. Stocker DDS
Contributor: D. A. Stocker M. Ed.
Contributor: Dr. N. Wyatt
Contributor: Sheila M. Hynes, MES York, BA (Hons)
Contributor: Elizabeta Petrovic MSc (Mathematics)

Published by
Complete Test Preparation Inc.
921 Foul Bay Rd.
Victoria BC Canada V8S 4H9
Visit us on the web at http://www.test-preparation.ca
Printed in the USA

Contact us at feedback@test-preparation.ca

Customizing and White Label Service

Have your logo and school name on the front cover in a special edition produced for your school or institution. Visit http://test-preparation.ca/customization.html or please contact us for details at sales@test-preparation.ca

Feedback

We welcome your feedback. Email us at feedback@test-preparation.ca with your comments and suggestions.   We carefully review all suggestions and often incorporate reader suggestions into upcoming versions. As a Print on Demand Publisher, we update our products frequently.

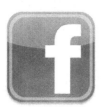

Find us on Facebook

Go to www.facebook.com/CompleteTestPreparation

Contents

Getting Started

CONGRATULATIONS! By deciding to take the Registered Nursing Program (PAX RN) Exam, you have taken the first step toward a great future! Of course, there is no point in taking this important examination unless you intend to do your very best in order to earn the highest grade you possibly can. That means getting yourself organized and discovering the best approaches, methods and strategies to master the material. Yes, that will require real effort and dedication on your part but if you are willing to focus your energy and devote the study time necessary, before you know it you will be opening that letter of acceptance to the school of your dreams.

We know that taking on a new endeavour can be a little scary, and it is easy to feel unsure of where to begin. That's where we come in. This study guide is designed to help you improve your test-taking skills, show you a few tricks of the trade and increase both your competency and confidence.

The Registered Nursing Program PAX RN Exam

The PAX RN Modules are: Mathematics, Verbal Ability (Reading Comprehension and Vocabulary), and Science which includes, Biology, Chemistry, Physics, Basic Scientific principals and Earth Science.

While we seek to make our guide as comprehensive as possible, it is important to note that like all entrance exams, the PAX RN Exam might be adjusted at some future point. New material might be added, or content that is no longer relevant or applicable might be removed. It is always a good idea to give the materials you receive when you register to take the PAX RN a careful review.

How this study guide is organized

This study guide is divided into four sections. The first section, Self-Assessments, which will help you recognize your areas of strength and weaknesses. This will be a boon when it comes to managing your study time most efficiently; there is not much point of focusing on material you have already got firmly under control. Instead, taking the self-assessments will show you where that time could be much better spent. In this area you will begin with a few questions to quickly evaluate your understanding of material that is likely to appear on the PAX RN. If you do poorly in certain areas, simply work carefully through those sections in the tutorials and then try the self-assessment again.

The second section, Tutorials, offers information in each of the content areas, as well as strategies to help you master that material. The tutorials are not intended to be a complete course, but cover general principals. If you find that you do not understand the tutorials, it is recommended that you seek out additional instruction. Most Universities recommend student take introductory courses in Math, English and Science before taking the PAX RN.

Third, we offer two sets of practice test questions, similar to those on the PAX RN Exam. Again, we cover all modules, so make sure to check with your school!

In addition to all these materials, the last three chapters give you important information on how to answer multiple choice questions, how to prepare for a test, and how to take a test.

The PAX RN Study Plan

Now that you have made the decision to take the PAX RN, it is time to get started. Before you do another thing, you will need to figure out a plan of attack. The very best study tip is to start early! The longer the time period you devote to regular study practice, the more likely you will be to retain the material and be able to access it quickly. If you thought that 1x20 is the same as 2x10, guess what? It really is not, when it comes to study time. Reviewing material for just an hour per day over the course of 20 days is far better than studying for two hours a day for only 10 days. The more often you revisit a particular piece of information, the better you will know it. Not only will your grasp and understanding be better, but your ability to reach into your brain and quickly and efficiently pull out the tidbit you need, will be greatly enhanced as well.

The great Chinese scholar and philosopher Confucius believed that true knowledge could be defined as knowing both what you know and what you do not know. The first step in preparing for the PAX RN Exam is to assess your strengths and weaknesses. You may already have an idea of what you know and what you do not know, but evaluating yourself using our Self- Assessment modules for each of the three areas, Math, Science and Verbal Ability, will clarify the details.

Making a Study Schedule

In order to make your study time most productive you will need to develop a study plan. The purpose of the plan is to organize all the bits of pieces of information in such a way that you will not feel overwhelmed. Rome was not built in a day, and learning everything you will need to know in order to pass the PAX RN Exam is going to take time, too. Arranging the material you need to learn into manageable chunks is the best way to go. Each study session should make you feel as though you have succeeded in accomplishing your goal, and your goal is simply to learn what you planned to learn during that particular session. Try to organize the content in such a way that each study session builds upon previous ones. That way, you will retain the information, be better able to access it, and review the previous bits and pieces at the same time.

Self-assessment

The Best Study Tip! The very best study tip is to start early! The longer you study regularly, the more you will retain and 'learn' the material. Studying for 1 hour per day for 20 days is far better than studying for 2 hours for 10 days.

What don't you know?

The first step is to assess your strengths and weaknesses. You may already have an idea of where your weaknesses are, or you can take our Self-assessment modules for each of the areas, Math, Science and Verbal Ability.

Exam Component	Rate 1 to 5
Verbal Ability	
Paragraph & Passage Comprehension	
Vocabulary	
Math	
Fractions, Decimals, Percent	
Word Problems	
Percent	
Median and Mode	
Scientific Notation	
Quadratics and Polynomials	
Speed and Momentum	
Basic Algebra	
Science	
Biology	
Physics	
Earth Science	
Chemistry	

Making a Study Schedule

The key to making a study plan is to divide the material you need to learn into manageable size and learn it, while at the same time reviewing the material that you already know.

Using the table above, any scores of 3 or below, you need to spend time learning, going over and practicing this subject area. A score of 4 means you need to review the material, but you don't have to spend time re-learning. A score of 5 and you are OK with just an occasional review before the exam.

A score of 0 or 1 means you really need to work on this area and should allocate the most time and the highest priority. Some students prefer a 5-day plan and others a 10-day plan. It also depends on how much time you have until the exam.

Here is an example of a 5-day plan based on an example from the table above:

Fractions: 1 Study 1 hour everyday – review on last day
Biology: 3 Study 1 hour for 2 days then ½ hour a day, then review
Vocabulary: 4 Review every second day
Word Problems: 2 Study 1 hour on the first day – then ½ hour everyday
Reading Comprehension: 5 Review for ½ hour every other day
Algebra: 5 Review for ½ hour every other day
Chemistry: 5 very confident – review a few times.

Based on this, here is a sample study plan:

Day	Subject	Time
Monday		
Study	Fractions	1 hour
Study	Word Problems	1 hour
	½ hour break	
Study	Biology	1 hour
Review	Chemistry	½ hour
Tuesday		
Study	Fractions	1 hour
Study	Word Problems	½ hour
	½ hour break	
Study	Decimals	½ hour
Review	Vocabulary	½ hour
Review	Grammar	½ hour

Wednesday		
Study	Fractions	1 hour
Study	Word Problems	½ hour
	½ hour break	
Study	Biology	½ hour
Review	Chemistry	½ hour
Thursday		
Study	Fractions	½ hour
Study	Word Problems	½ hour
Review	Biology	½ hour
	½ hour break	
Review	Grammar	½ hour
Review	Vocabulary	½ hour
Friday		
Review	Fractions	½ hour
Review	Word Problems	½ hour
Review	Biology	½ hour
	½ hour break	
Review	Vocabulary	½ hour
Review	Grammar	½ hour

Verbal Ability

THIS SECTION CONTAINS A SELF-ASSESSMENT AND READING TUTORIAL. The Tutorials are designed to familiarize general principals and the self-assessment contains general questions similar to the reading questions likely to be on the PAX RN exam, but are not intended to be identical to the exam questions. Many Universities recommend that students take an introductory courses before taking the PAX RN Exam. The tutorials are not designed to be a complete reading course, and it is assumed that students have some familiarity with Verbal Ability questions. If you do not understand parts of the tutorial, or find the tutorial difficult, it is recommended that you seek out additional instruction.

Tour of the PAX RN Reading Content

The PAX RN reading section has 47 questions that must be answered in 60 minutes. Below is a more detailed list of the types of reading questions that generally appear on the PAX RN. Make sure you understand all of these points at a very minimum.

- Drawing logical conclusions

- Identifying main ideas

- Meaning in context

- Distinguish fact from opinions

- Making inferences

- Identifying tone and purpose

- Summarizing

The questions below are not exactly the same as you will find on the PAX RN - that would be too easy! And nobody knows what the questions will be and they change all the time. Mostly the changes consist of substituting new questions for old, but the changes can be new question formats or styles, changes to the number of questions in each section, changes to the time limits for each section and combining sections. Below are general reading questions that cover the same areas as the PAX RN. So while the format and exact wording of the questions may differ slightly, and change from year to year, if you can answer the questions below, you will have no problem with the verbal ability section of the PAX RN.

Reading Self-Assessment

The purpose of the self-assessment is:

- Identify your strengths and weaknesses.

- Develop your personalized study plan (above)

- Get accustomed to the PAX RN format

- Extra practice – the self-assessments are almost a full 3rd practice test!

- Provide a baseline score for preparing your study schedule.

Since this is a Self-assessment, and depending on how confident you are with Verbal Ability, timing is optional. The PAX RN has 80 reading questions including vocabulary. The self-assessment has 40 questions, so allow about 45 minutes to complete this assessment.

Once complete, use the table below to assess your understanding of the content, and prepare your study schedule described in chapter 1.

80% - 100%	Excellent – you have mastered the content
60 – 79%	Good. You have a working knowledge. Even though you can just pass this section, you may want to review the tutorials and do some extra practice to see if you can improve your mark.
40% - 59%	Below Average. You do not understand the Verbal Ability problems. Review the tutorials, and retake this quiz again in a few days, before proceeding to the rest of the study guide.
Less than 40%	Poor. You have a very limited understanding of the Verbal Ability problems. Please review the tutorials, and retake this quiz again in a few days, before proceeding to the rest of the study guide.

Verbal Ability Self-Assessment Answer Sheet

1.	A B C D	11.	A B C D	21.	A B C D	31.	A B C D
2.	A B C D	12.	A B C D	22.	A B C D	32.	A B C D
3.	A B C D	13.	A B C D	23.	A B C D	33.	A B C D
4.	A B C D	14.	A B C D	24.	A B C D	34.	A B C D
5.	A B C D	15.	A B C D	25.	A B C D	35.	A B C D
6.	A B C D	16.	A B C D	26.	A B C D	36.	A B C D
7.	A B C D	17.	A B C D	27.	A B C D	37.	A B C D
8.	A B C D	18.	A B C D	28.	A B C D	38.	A B C D
9.	A B C D	19.	A B C D	29.	A B C D	39.	A B C D
10.	A B C D	20.	A B C D	30.	A B C D	40.	A B C D

Questions 1 – 4 refer to the following passage.

The Immune System

An immune system is a system of biological structures and processes that protects against disease by identifying and killing pathogens and other threats. The immune system can detect a wide variety of agents, from viruses to parasitic worms, and distinguish them from the organism's own healthy cells and tissues. Detection is complicated as pathogens evolve rapidly to avoid the immune system defences, and successfully infect their hosts.

The human immune system consists of many types of proteins, cells, organs, and tissues, which interact in an elaborate and dynamic network. As part of this more complex immune response, the human immune system adapts over time to recognize specific pathogens more efficiently. This adaptation process is referred to as "adaptive immunity" or "acquired immunity" and creates immunological memory. Immunological memory created from a primary response to a specific pathogen, provides an enhanced response to future encounters with that same pathogen. This process of acquired immunity is the basis of vaccination. [1]

1. What can we infer from the first paragraph in this passage?

    a. When a person's body fights off the flu, this is the immune system in action

    b. When a person's immune system functions correctly, they avoid all sicknesses and injuries

    c. When a person's immune system is weak, a person will likely get a terminal disease

    d. When a person's body fights off a cold, this is the circulatory system in action

2. The immune system's primary function is to:

    a. Strengthen the bones

    b. Protect against disease

    c. Improve respiration

    d. Improve circulation

3. Based on the passage, what can we say about evolution's role in the immune system?

    a. Evolution of the immune system is an important factor in the immune system's efficiency

    b. Evolution causes a person to die, thus killing the pathogen

    c. Evolution plays no known role in immunity

    d. The least evolved earth species have better immunity

4. Acquired immunity is another term for what?

    a. White blood cells

    b. AIDS

    c. Adaptive immunity

    d. Disease

Questions 5 – 8 refer to the following passage.

White Blood Cells

White blood cells (WBCs), or leukocytes (also spelled "leucocytes"), are cells of the immune system that defend the body against both infectious disease and foreign material. Five different and diverse types of leukocytes exist, but they are all produced and derived from a powerful cell in the bone marrow known as a hematopoietic stem cell. Leukocytes are found throughout the body, including the blood and lymphatic system.

The number of WBCs in the blood is often an indicator of disease. There are normally between 4×10^9 and 1.1×10^{10} white blood cells in a liter of blood, making up approximately 1% of blood in a healthy adult. The physical properties of white blood cells, such as volume, conductivity, and granularity, changes due to the presence of immature cells, or malignant cells.

The name white blood cell derives from the fact that after processing a blood sample in a centrifuge, the white cells are typically a thin, white layer of nucleated cells. The scientific term leukocyte directly reflects this description, derived from Greek leukos (white), and kytos (cell). [2]

5. What can we infer from the first paragraph in this selection?

    a. Red blood cells are not as important as white blood cells

    b. White blood cells are the culprits in most infectious diseases

    c. White blood cells are essential to fight off infectious diseases

    d. Red blood cells are essential to fight off infectious diseases

6. What can we say about the number of white blood cells in a liter of blood?

    a. They make up about 1% of a healthy adult's blood

    b. There are 10^{10} WBCs in a healthy adult's blood

    c. The number varies according to age

    d. They are a thin white layer of nucleated cells

7. What is a more scientific term for "white blood cell"?

    a. Red blood cell

    b. Anthrocyte

    c. Leukocyte

    d. Leukemia

8. Can the number of leukocytes indicate cancer?

    a. Yes, the white blood cell count can indicate disease.

    b. No, the white blood cell count is not a reliable indicator.

    c. Yes, disease can indicate a high white cell count.

    d. None of the choices are correct.

Questions 9 - 10 refer to the following passage.

Thunderstorms I

Warm air is less dense than cool air, so warm air rises within cooler air like a hot air balloon or warm water in an ocean current. Clouds form as warm air carrying moisture rises. As the warm air rises, it cools, and the moist water vapor begins to condense. This releases energy that keeps the air warmer than its surroundings, and as a result, continues to rise. If enough instability is present in the atmosphere, this process will continue long enough for cumulonimbus clouds to form, which support lightning and thunder. All thunderstorms, regardless of type, go through three stages: the cumulus stage, the mature stage, and the dissipation stage. Depending on the conditions in the atmosphere, these three stages can take anywhere from 20 minutes to several hours. [3]

9. This passage tells us

    a. Warm air is denser than cool air

    b. All thunderstorms go through three stages

    c. Thunderstorms may occur without clouds present

    d. The stages of a thunderstorm conclude within just a few minutes

10. When warm air rises through colder air, it results in

    a. Evaporation

    b. Humidity

    c. Clear skies

    d. Condensation

Questions 10 – 12 refer to the following passage.

Vice President Johnson, Mr. Speaker, Mr. Chief Justice, President Eisenhower, Vice President Nixon, President Truman, reverend clergy, fellow citizens:

We observe today not a victory of party, but a celebration of freedom -- symbolizing an end, as well as a beginning -- signifying renewal, as well as change. For I have sworn before you and Almighty God the same solemn oath our forebears prescribed nearly a century and three-quarters ago.

The world is very different now. For man holds in his mortal hands the power to abolish all forms of human poverty and all forms of human life. And yet the same revolutionary beliefs for which our forebears fought are still at issue around the globe -- the belief that the rights of man come not from the generosity of the state, but from the hand of God.

We dare not forget today that we are the heirs of that first revolution. Let the word go forth from this time and place, to friend and foe alike, that the torch has been passed to a new generation of Americans -- born in this century, tempered by war, disciplined by a hard and bitter peace, proud of our ancient heritage, and unwilling to witness or permit the slow undoing of those human rights to which this nation has always been committed, and to which we are committed today at home and around the world.

Let every nation know, whether it wishes us well or ill, that we shall pay any price, bear any burden, meet any hardship, support any friend, oppose any foe, to assure the survival and the success of liberty.

This much we pledge -- and more.

John F. Kennedy Inaugural Address delivered 20 January 1961

11. What is the tone of this speech?

    a. Triumphant

    b. Optimistic

    c. Threatening

    d. Gloating

12. Which of the following is an opinion?

a. The world is very different now.

b. For man holds in his mortal hands the power to abolish all forms of human poverty and all forms of human life.

c. We dare not forget today that we are the heirs of that first revolution

d. For I have sworn before you and Almighty God the same solemn oath our forebears prescribed nearly a century and three-quarters ago.

Questions 13 – 15 refer to the following passage.

How To Get A Good Nights Sleep

Sleep is just as essential for healthy living as water, air and food. Sleep allows the body to rest and replenish depleted energy levels. Sometimes we may for various reasons experience difficulty sleeping which has a serious effect on our health. Those who have prolonged sleeping problems are facing a serious medical condition and should see a qualified doctor as soon as possible for help. Here is simple guide that can help you sleep better at night.

Try to create a natural pattern of waking up and sleeping around the same time every-day. This means avoiding going to bed too early and oversleeping past your usual wake up time. Going to bed and getting up at radically different times everyday confuses your body clock. Try to establish a natural rhythm as much as you can.

Exercises and a bit of physical activity can help you sleep better at night. If you are having problem sleeping, try to be as active as you can during the day. If you are tired from physical activity, falling asleep is a natural and easy process for your body. If you remain inactive during the day, you will find it harder to sleep properly at night. Try walking, jogging, swimming or simple stretches as you get close to your bed time.

Afternoon naps are great to refresh you during the day, but they may also keep you awake at night. If you feel sleepy during the day, get up, take a walk and get busy to keep from sleeping. Stretching is a good way to increase blood flow to the brain and keep you alert so that you don't sleep during the day. This will help you sleep better night.

A warm bath or a glass of milk in the evening can help your body relax and prepare for sleep. A cold bath will wake you up and keep you up for several hours. Also avoid eating too late before bed.

13. How would you describe this sentence?

    a. A recommendation

    b. An opinion

    c. A fact

    d. A diagnosis

14. Which of the following is an alternative title for this article?

    a. Exercise and a good night's sleep

    b. Benefits of a good night's sleep

    c. Tips for a good night's sleep

    d. Lack of sleep is a serious medical condition

15. Which of the following can not be inferred from this article?

    a. Biking is helpful for getting a good night's sleep

    b. Mental activity is helpful for getting a good night's sleep

    c. Eating bedtime snacks is not recommended

    d. Getting up at the same time is helpful for a good night's sleep

Part II – Vocabulary

16. Choose the noun that means, self evident or clear obvious truth.

    a. Truism

    b. Catharsis

    c. Libertine

    d. Tractable

17. Choose the best definition for: virago

    a. A loud domineering woman

    b. A quiet woman

    c. A load domineering Man

    d. A quiet man

18. When Joe broke his _____ in a skiing accident, his entire leg was in a cast.

    a. Ankle

    b. Humerus

    c. Wrist

    d. Femur

19. Select another word for the underlined word in the sentence below.

At first I thought she was very rude and boorish, but when I talked to her again she was very <u>genteel.</u>

    a. Chivalrous

    b. Hilarious

    c. Civilized

    d. Governance

20. Choose an adjective that means corrupted, impure.

    a. Adulterate

    b. Harbor

    c. Infuriate

    d. Inculcate

21. Select another word for the underlined word in the sentence below.

Her business success showed that she was very <u>shrewd</u>.

    a. Slow

    b. astute

    c. Ignorant

    d. Heinous

22. Choose an adjective that means, beyond what is obvious or evident.

    a. Ulterior

    b. Sybarite

    c. Torsion

    d. Trenchant

23. Choose a noun that means, homeless child or stray.

    a. Elegy

    b. Waif

    c. Martyr

    d. Palaver

24. Select another word for the under-lined word in the sentence below.

His inheritance was very large - a _princely_ sum!

    a. Minor
    b. Tolerable
    c. Large
    d. Pittance

25. What is the best definition of depre-cate?

    a. Approve
    b. Indifference
    c. Disapprove
    d. None of the above

26. Choose the best definition for suc-cor.

    a. To suck on
    b. To hate
    c. To like
    d. Give help of assistance

27. Select the synonym of conspicuous.

    a. Important
    b. Prominent
    c. Beautiful
    d. Convincing

28. Select the noun that means eager-ness and enthusiasm.

    a. Alacrity
    b. Happiness
    c. Donator
    d. Marital

29. Fill in the blank.

After Lisa's aunt had her tenth child, Lisa found that she had more than twenty _____.

    a. Uncles
    b. Friends
    c. Stepsisters
    d. Cousins

30. Select the word that means benevo-lence.

    a. Happiness
    b. Courage
    c. Kindness
    d. Loyalty

31. Select the verb that means, to make less severe.

    a. Suspense
    b. Alleviate
    c. Ingrate
    d. Action

32. What is the name of one who gives a gift or who gives money to a charity organization?

    a. Captain
    b. Benefactor
    c. Source
    d. Teacher

33. What is another word for subordinate, or person of lesser rank or authority?

    a. Palliate

    b. Plebeian

    c. Underling

    d. Expiate

34. Choose the best definition of specious.

    a. Logical

    b. Illogical

    c. Emotional

    d. 2 species

35. Choose the best definition of proscribe.

    a. Welcome

    b. Write a prescription

    c. Banish

    d. Give a diagnosis

36. Fill in the blank.

When Craig's dog was struck by a car, he rushed his pet to the _____.

    a. Emergency room

    b. Doctor

    c. Veterinarian

    d. Podiatrist

37. Select another word for the underlined word in the sentence below. She never made a mistake - her performance was always <u>impeccable</u>.

    a. Charming

    b. Flattering

    c. Perfect

    d. Impervious

38. Select the synonym of boisterous.

    a. Loud

    b. Soft

    c. Gentle

    d. Warm

39. Select the adjective that means hidden, secret, disguised.

    a. Accustomed

    b. Covert

    c. Hide

    d. Carriage

40. Select the verb that means straightforward, open and sincere.

    a. Lawful

    b. Candid

    c. True

    d. Lawful

Answer Key

1. A

The passage does not mention the flu specifically, however we know the flu is a pathogen (A bacterium, virus, or other microorganism that can cause disease). Therefore, we can infer, when a person's body fights off the flu, this is the immune system in action.

2. B

The immune system's primary function is to protect against disease.

3. A

The passage refers to evolution of the immune system being important for efficiency. In paragraph three, there is a discussion of adaptive and acquired immunity, where the immune system "remembers" pathogens.

We can conclude, evolution of the immune system is an important factor in the immune system's efficiency.

4. C

This is taken directly from the passage. Acquired immunity is another term for adaptive immunity.

5. C

We can infer white blood cells are essential to fight off infectious diseases, from the passage, "cells of the immune system that defend the body against both infectious disease and foreign material."

6. A

We can say the number of white blood cells in a liter of blood make up about 1% of a healthy adult's blood. This is a fact-based question that is easy and fast to answer. The question asks about a percentage. You can quickly and easily scan to passage for the percent sign, or the word percent and find the answer.

7. C

A more scientific term for "white blood cell" is leukocyte, from the first paragraph, first sentence of the passage.

8. A

The white blood cell count can indicate disease (cancer). We know this from the last sentence of paragraph two, "The physical properties of white blood cells, such as volume, conductivity, and granularity, changes due to the presence of immature cells, or malignant cells."

9. B

All thunderstorms will go through three stages. This is taken directly from the text, "All thunderstorms, regardless of type, go through three stages: the cumulus stage, the mature stage, and the dissipation stage."

10. D

Condensation. From the passage, "As the warm air rises, it cools, and the moist water vapor begins to condense."

11. A

This is a triumphant speech where President Kennedy is celebrating his victory.

12. C

The statement, "We dare not forget today that we are the heirs of that first revolution" is an opinion.

13. A

The sentence is a recommendation.

14. C

Tips for a good night's sleep is the best alternative title for this article.

15. B

Mental activity is helpful for a good night's sleep is can not be inferred from this article.

16. A

Truism: n. self evident or clear obvious

truth.

17. A
Virago: Given to undue belligerence or ill manner at the slightest provocation; a shrew, a termagant.

18. D
Femur: n. The bone of the thigh or upper hind limb, articulating at the hip and the knee.

19. C
Genteel: Polite and well-mannered. Stylish or elegant. Aristocratic

20. A
Adulterate: v. To render (something) poorer in quality by adding another substance, typically an inferior one.

21. B
Shrewd: showing clever resourcefulness in practical matters, artful, tricky or cunning, streetwise, knowledgeable.

22. A
Ulterior: adj. beyond what is obvious or evident.

23. B
Waif: n. homeless child or stray.

24. C
Princely: adj. In the manner of a royal prince's conduct; large or grand.

25. C
Deprecate: v. To belittle or express disapproval of.

26. D
Succor: n. Aid, assistance or relief given to one in distress; ministration.

27. B
Prominent: adj. Important, famous.

28. A
Alacrity: adj. Eagerness; liveliness; enthusiasm.

29. D
Cousins

30. C
Benevolent: adj. Well meaning and kindly.

31. B
Alleviate: v. To make less severe, as a pain or difficulty.

32. B
Benefactor: n. Somebody who gives one a gift. Usually refers to someone who gives money to a charity or another form of organization.

33. C
Underling: n. subordinate of lesser rank or authority.

34. B
Specious: adj. Seemingly well-reasoned or factual, but actually fallacious or insincere; strongly held but false.

35. C
Proscribe: v. To forbid or denounce.

36. C
Veterinarian: n. A person qualified to treat diseased or injured animals.

37. C
Impeccable: adj. Perfect, without faults, flaws or errors.

38. A
Boisterous: adj. Noisy, energetic, and cheerful; rowdy.

39. B
Covert: adj. Partially hidden, disguised, secret, surreptitious.

40. B
Candid: adj. Straightforward, open and sincere.

Help with Reading Comprehension

At first sight, reading comprehension tests look challenging especially if you are given long essays to answer only two to three questions. While reading, you might notice your attention wandering, or feeling sleepy. Do not be discouraged because there are various tactics and long range strategies that make comprehending even long, boring essays easier.

Your friends before your foes. It is always best to tackle essays or passages with familiar subjects rather than those with unfamiliar ones. This approach applies the same logic as tackling easy questions before hard ones. Skip passages that do not interest you and leave them for later when there is more time left.

Don't use 'special' reading techniques. This is not the time for speed-reading or anything like that – just plain ordinary reading – not too slow and not too fast.

Read through the entire passage and the questions before you do anything. Many students try reading the questions first and then looking for answers in the passage thinking this approach is more efficient. What these students do not realize is that it is often hard to navigate in unfamiliar roads. If you do not familiarize yourself with the passage first, looking for answers become not only time-consuming but also dangerous because you might miss the context of the answer you are looking for. If you read the questions first you will only confuse yourself and lose valuable time.

Familiarize yourself with reading comprehension questions. If you are familiar with the common types of reading comprehension questions, you are able to take note of important parts of the passage, saving time. There are six major kinds of reading comprehension questions.

- **Main Idea**- Questions that ask for the central thought or significance of the passage.

- **Specific Details** - Questions that asks for explicitly stated ideas.

- **Drawing Inferences** - Questions that ask for a statement's intended meaning.

- **Tone or Attitude** - Questions that test your ability to sense the emotional state of the author.

- **Context Meaning** – Questions that ask for the meaning of a word depending on the context.

- **Technique** – Questions that ask for the method of organization or the writing style of the author.

Read. Read. Read. The best preparation for reading comprehension tests is always to read, read and read. If you are not used to reading lengthy passages, you will probably lose concentration. Increase your attention span by making a habit out of reading.

Reading Comprehension tests become less daunting when you have trained yourself to read and understand fast. Always remember that it is easier to understand passages you are interested in. Do not read through passages hastily. Make mental notes of ideas that you think might be asked.

Reading Comprehension Strategy

When facing the reading comprehension section of a standardized test, you need a strategy to be successful. You want to keep several steps in mind:

• First, make a note of the time and the number of sections. Time your work accordingly. Typically, four to five minutes per section is sufficient. Second, read the directions for each selection thoroughly before beginning (and listen well to any additional verbal instructions, as they will often clarify obscure or confusing written guidelines). You must know exactly how to do what you're about to do!

• Now you're ready to begin reading the selection. Read the passage carefully, noting significant characters or events on a scratch sheet of paper or underlining on the test sheet. Many students find making a basic list in the margins helpful. Quickly jot down or underline one-word summaries of characters, notable happenings, numbers, or key ideas. This will help you better retain information and focus wandering thoughts. Remember, however, that your main goal in doing this is to find the information that answers the questions. Even if you find the passage interesting, remember your goal and work fast but stay on track.

• Now read the question and all of the choices. Now you have read the passage, have a general idea of the main ideas, and have marked the important points. Read the question and all of the choices. Never choose an answer without reading them all! Questions are often designed to confuse – stay focussed and clear. Usually the answer choices will focus on one or two facts or inferences from the passage. Keep these clear in your mind.

• Search for the answer. With a very general idea of what the different choices are, go back to the passage and scan for the relevant information. Watch for big words, unusual or unique words. These make your job easier as you can scan the text for the particular word.

• Mark the Answer. Now you have the key information the question is looking for. Go back to the question, quickly scan the choices and mark the correct one.

Understand and practice the different types of standardized reading comprehension tests. See the list above for the different types. Typically, there will be several questions dealing with facts from the selection, a couple more inference questions dealing with logical consequences of those facts, and periodically an application-oriented question surfaces to force you to make connections with what you already know. Some students prefer to answer the questions as listed, and feel classifying the question and then ordering is wasting precious time. Other students prefer to answer the different types of questions in order of how easy or difficult they are. The choice is yours and do whatever works for you. If you want to try answering in order of difficulty, here is a recommended order, answer fact questions first; they're easily found within the passage. Tackle inference problems next, after re-reading the question(s) as many times as you need to. Application or 'best guess' questions usually take the longest, so save them for last.

Use the practice tests to try out both ways of answering and see what works for you.

For more help with reading comprehension, see Multiple Choice Secrets.

Help with Building your Vocabulary

Vocabulary tests can be daunting when you think of the enormous number of words that might come up in the exam. As the exam date draws near, your anxiety will grow because you know that no matter how many words you memorize, chances are, you will still remember so few. Here are some tips which you can use to hurdle the big words that may come up in your exam without having to open the dictionary and memorize all the words known to humankind.

Build up and tear apart the big words. Big words, like many other things, are composed of small parts. Some words are made up of many other words. A man who lifts weights for example, is a weight lifter. Words are also made up of word parts called prefixes, suffixes and roots. Often times, we can see the relationship of different words through these parts. A person who is skilled with both hands is ambidextrous. A word with double meaning is ambiguous. A person with two conflicting emotions is ambivalent. Two words with synonymous meanings often have the same root. Bio, a root word derived from Latin is used in words like biography meaning to write about a person's life, and biology meaning the study of living organisms.

- **Words with double meanings.** Did you know that the word husband not only means a man married to a woman, but also thrift or frugality? Sometimes, words have double meanings. The dictionary meaning, or the denotation of a word is sometimes different from the way we use it or its connotation.

- **Read widely, read deeply and read daily.** The best way to expand your vocabulary is to familiarize yourself with as many words as possible through reading. By reading, you are able to remember words in a proper context and thus, remember its meaning or at the very least, its use. Reading widely would help you get acquainted with words you may never use every day. This is the best strategy without doubt. However, if you are studying for an exam next week, or even tomorrow, it isn't much help! Below you will find a range of different ways to learn new words quickly and efficiently.

- **Remember.** Always remember that big words are easy to understand when divided into smaller parts, and the smaller words will often have several other meanings aside from the one you already know. Below is an extensive list of root or stem words, followed by one hundred questions to help you learn word stems.

Here are suggested effective ways to help you improve your vocabulary.

Be Committed To Learning New Words. To improve your vocabulary you need to make a commitment to learn new words. Commit to learning at least a word or two a day. You can also get new words by reading books, poems, stories, plays and magazines. Expose yourself to more language to increase the number of new words that you learn.

- **Learn Practical Vocabulary**. As much as possible, learn vocabulary that is associated with what you do and that you can use regularly. For example learn words related to your profession or hobby. Learn as much vocabulary as you can in your favorite subjects.

- **Use New Words Frequently**. As soon as you learn a new word start using it and do so frequently. Repeat it when you are alone and try to use the word as often as you can with people you talk to. You can also use flashcards to practice new words that you learn.

- **Learn the Proper Usage.** If you do not understand the proper usage, look it up and make sure you have it right.

- **Use a Dictionary**. When reading textbooks, novels or assigned readings, keep the dictionary nearby. Also learn how to use online dictionaries and WORD dictionary. As soon as you come across a new word, check for its meaning. If you cannot do so immediately, then you should right it down and check it as soon as possible. This will help you understand what the word means and exactly how best to use it.

- **Learn Word Roots, Prefixes and Suffixes.** English words are usually derived from suffixes, prefixes and roots, which come from Latin, French or Greek. Learning the root or origin of a word helps you easily understand the meaning of the word and other words that are derived from the root. Generally, if you learn the meaning of one root word, you will understand two or three words. See our List of Stem Words below. This is a great two-for-one strategy. Most prefixes, suffixes, roots and stems are used in two, three or more words, so if you know the root, prefix or suffix, you can guess the meaning of many words.

- **Synonyms and Antonyms**. Most words in the English language have two or three (at least) synonyms and antonyms. For example, "big," in the most common usage, has about seventy-five synonyms and an equal number of antonyms. Understanding the relationships between these words and how they all fit together gives your brain a framework, which makes them easier to learn, remember and recall.

- **Use Flash Cards**. Flash cards are one of the best ways to memorize things. They can be used anywhere and anytime, so you can make use of odd free moments waiting for the bus or waiting in line. Make your own or buy commercially prepared flash cards, and keep them with you all the time.

- **Make word lists.** Learning vocabulary, like learning many things, requires repetition. Keep a new words journal in a separate section or separate notebook. Add any words that you look up in the dictionary, as well as from word lists. Review your word lists regularly.

Photocopying or printing off word lists from the Internet or handouts is not the same. Actually writing out the word and a few notes on the definition is an important process for imprinting the word in your brain. Writing out the word and definition in your New Word Journal, forces you to concentrate and focus on the new word. Hitting PRINT or pushing the button on the photocopier does not do the same thing.

Notice the verbs in bold in the examples above. They are encircling the subjects of each sentence rather than following them. This is inverse word order.

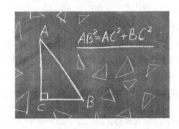

Mathematics

THIS SECTION CONTAINS A SELF-ASSESSMENT AND MATH TUTORIALS. The Tutorials are designed to familiarize general principals and the self-assessment contains general questions similar to the reading questions likely to be on the PAX RN exam, but are not intended to be identical to the exam questions. Many Universities recommend that students take an introductory courses before taking the PAX RN Exam. The tutorials are not designed to be a complete mathematics course, and it is assumed that students have some familiarity with math questions. If you do not understand parts of the tutorial, or find the tutorial difficult, it is recommended that you seek out additional instruction.

Tour of the PAX RN Mathematics Content

The PAX RN reading section has 50 questions. Below is a more detailed list of the types of math questions that generally appear on the PAX RN. Make sure you understand all of these points at a very minimum.

- Basic operations - adding subtracting, multiplying and dividing whole numbers

- Square root

- Prime factors

- Median and mode

- Exponents

- Word problems

- Simple geometry

- IQ questions

- Operations with polynomials

- Quadratics

- Ratio and proportion

- Fractions, decimals and percent

- Speed, acceleration and momentum

The questions below are not exactly the same as you will find on the PAX RN - that would be too easy! And nobody knows what the questions will be and they change all the time. Mostly the changes consist of substituting new questions for old, but the changes can be new question formats or styles, changes to the number of questions in each section, changes to the time limits for each section and combining sections. Below are general math questions that cover the same areas as the PAX RN. So while the format and exact wording of the questions may differ slightly, and change from year to year, if you can answer the questions below, you will have no problem with the math section of the PAX RN.

Math Self-Assessment

The purpose of the self-assessment is:

- Identify your strengths and weaknesses.

- Develop your personalized study plan (above)

- Get accustomed to the PAX RN format

- Extra practice – the self-assessments are almost a full 3rd practice test!

- Provide a baseline score for preparing your study schedule.

Since this is a Self-assessment, and depending on how confident you are with math, timing is optional. The PAX RN has 50 reading questions to be answered in 50 minutes. The self-assessment has 50 questions, so allow 50 minutes to complete this assessment.

Once complete, use the table below to assess your understanding of the content, and prepare your study schedule described in chapter 1.

80% - 100%	Excellent – you have mastered the content
60 – 79%	Good. You have a working knowledge. Even though you can just pass this section, you may want to review the tutorials and do some extra practice to see if you can improve your mark.
40% - 59%	Below Average. You do not understand the math problems. Review the tutorials, and retake this quiz again in a few days, before proceeding to the rest of the Practice Test.
Less than 40%	Poor. You have a very limited understanding of math. Please review the tutorials, and retake this quiz again in a few days, before proceeding to the rest of the study guide.

Math Self-Assessment Answer Sheet

1. (A) (B) (C) (D)
2. (A) (B) (C) (D)
3. (A) (B) (C) (D)
4. (A) (B) (C) (D)
5. (A) (B) (C) (D)
6. (A) (B) (C) (D)
7. (A) (B) (C) (D)
8. (A) (B) (C) (D)
9. (A) (B) (C) (D)
10. (A) (B) (C) (D)
11. (A) (B) (C) (D)
12. (A) (B) (C) (D)
13. (A) (B) (C) (D)
14. (A) (B) (C) (D)
15. (A) (B) (C) (D)
16. (A) (B) (C) (D)
17. (A) (B) (C) (D)

18. (A) (B) (C) (D)
19. (A) (B) (C) (D)
20. (A) (B) (C) (D)
21. (A) (B) (C) (D)
22. (A) (B) (C) (D)
23. (A) (B) (C) (D)
24. (A) (B) (C) (D)
25. (A) (B) (C) (D)
26. (A) (B) (C) (D)
27. (A) (B) (C) (D)
28. (A) (B) (C) (D)
29. (A) (B) (C) (D)
30. (A) (B) (C) (D)
31. (A) (B) (C) (D)
32. (A) (B) (C) (D)
33. (A) (B) (C) (D)
34. (A) (B) (C) (D)

35. (A) (B) (C) (D)
36. (A) (B) (C) (D)
37. (A) (B) (C) (D)
38. (A) (B) (C) (D)
39. (A) (B) (C) (D)
40. (A) (B) (C) (D)
41. (A) (B) (C) (D)
42. (A) (B) (C) (D)
43. (A) (B) (C) (D)
44. (A) (B) (C) (D)
45. (A) (B) (C) (D)
46. (A) (B) (C) (D)
47. (A) (B) (C) (D)
48. (A) (B) (C) (D)
49. (A) (B) (C) (D)
50. (A) (B) (C) (D)

Mathematics Self-Assessment

Decimals, Fractions and Percent

1. A person earns $25000 per month and pays $9000 income tax per year. The Government increased income tax by 0.5% per month and his monthly earning was raised $11000. How much more income tax does he pay per month?

    a. $1260

    b. $1050

    c. $750

    d. $510

2. A boy has 5 red balls, 3 white balls and 2 yellow balls. What percent of the balls are yellow?

    a. 2%

    b. 8%

    c. 20%

    d. 12%

3. There were some oranges in a basket, by adding 8/5 of these the total became 130. How many oranges were in the basket?

    a. 60

    b. 50

    c. 40

    d. 35

4. A 7 centimeter diameter pizza weighs 750 grams. If the diameter increased to 8.2 centimeters, how much more will it weigh?

    a. 279

    b. 129

    c. 185

    d. 305

5. A distributor purchased 550 kilogram potatoes for $165. He distributed all these at a rate of $6.4 per 20 kilograms to 15 shops, $3.4 per 10 kilograms to 12 shops and remaining at $1.8. If his distribution cost is $10 then what will be his profit?

    a. $10.40

    b. $13.60

    c. $14.90

    d. $23.40

6. Convert 0.45 to a fraction

    a. 7/20

    b. 7/45

    c. 9/20

    d. 3/20

7. How much pay does Mr. Johnson receive if he gives half of his pay to his family, $250 to his landlord, and has exactly 3/7 of his pay left after these expenses?

    a. $3600

    b. $3500

    c. $2800

    d. $1750

8. What is the square root of √225?

    a. 25

    b. 15

    c. 5

    d. 13

9. A man buys an item for $420 and has a balance of 3000.00. How much did he have before?

    a. $2,580

    b. $3,420

    c. $2,420

    d. $342

10. Divide 9.60 by 3.2

    a. 2.50

    b. 3

    c. 2.3

    d. 6.4

11. If a discount of 20% is given for a desk and Mark saves $45, how much did he pay for the desk?

    a. $225

    b. $160

    c. $180

    d. $210

12. 10% of p is also 1/5 of q. Which of the following is correct?

    a. p + p = q

    b. q/p = p

    c. p - q = q

    d. p/q = p

Basic Algebra

13. If X = 7 solve 3x + 5 – 2x

    a. x = 6

    b. x = 12

    c. x = 1

    d. x = 0

14. Solve the following equation 3(2x – 2) = 24 – 3x

    a. x = 24

    b. x = 9

    c. x = 10

    d. x = 3.33

15. Expand (x + 7) (x - 3)

    a. $x^2 + 4x – 21$

    b. x + 21

    c. 2x + 4 – 21

    d. 6x - 21

Mean Mode and Median

16. Find the mean of 100, 1050, 320, 600 and 150.

    a. 333

    b. 444

    c. 440

    d. 320

17. Find the median of the set of numbers – 1,2,3,4,5,6,7,8,9 and 10.

   a. 55

   b. 10

   c. 1

   d. 5.5

18. The following represents age distribution of students in an elementary class. Find the mode of the values – 7, 9, 10, 13, 11, 7, 9, 19, 12, 11, 9, 7, 9, 10, 11

   a. 7

   b. 9

   c. 10

   d. 11

Exponents

19. Express in 3^4 standard form

   a. 81

   b. 27

   c. 12

   d. 9

20. Simplify $4^3 + 2^4$

   a. 45

   b. 108

   c. 80

   d. 48

21. If a = 2 and y = 5, solve $xy^3 - x^3$

   a. 240

   b. 258

   c. 248

   d. 242

22. $X^3 \times X^2 =$

   a. 5^x

   b. x^{-5}

   c. x^{-1}

   d. x^5

23. Express 100000^0 in standard form.

   a. 1

   b. 0

   c. 100000

   d. 1000

24. Solve $\sqrt{144}$

   a. 14

   b. 72

   c. 24

   d. 12

Geometry

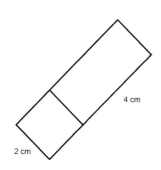

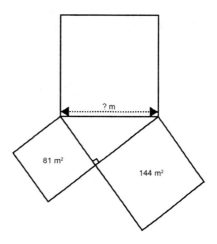

25. What is perimeter of the above shape?

    a. 12 cm
    b. 16 cm
    c. 6 cm
    d. 20 cm

27. What is the length of each side of the indicated square above?

    a. 10
    b. 15
    c. 20
    d. 5

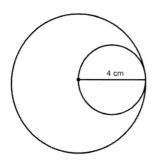

26. What is (area of large circle) - (area of small circle) in the figure above?

    a. 8 π cm²
    b. 10 π cm²
    c. 12 π cm²
    d. 16 π cm²

28. A bag contains 38 black balls and 42 white balls. What is the ratio of black balls to white?

    a. 9:11
    b. 1:3
    c. 19:21
    d. 11:9

29. The ratio of 8:5 = (?)%

    a. 75%
    b. 150%
    c. 175%
    d. 160%

30. 3 boys are asked to clean a surface that is 4 ft². If the portion is divided equally among the boys, what size will each of them clean?

    a. 1 ft 6 inches²

    b. 14 inches²

    c. 1 ft 2 inches²

    d. 16 inches²

31. Brian jogged 7 times around a circular track 75 meters in diameter. How much linear distance did he cover?

    a. 1250 meters

    b. 1650 meters

    c. 1450 meters

    d. 1725 meters

32. Consider the following population growth chart.

Country	Population 2000	Population 2005
Japan	122,251,000	128,057,000
China	1,145,195,000	1,341,335,000
United States	253,339,000	310,384,000
Indonesia	184,346,000	239,871,000

Which country is growing the fastest?

    a. Japan

    b. China

    c. United States

    d. Indonesia

Basic Math

33. 467 × 41 =

    a. 19,147

    b. 21,227

    c. 23,107

    d. 18,177

34. 1518 ÷ 27 =

    a. 54 r1

    b. 56 r6

    c. 55 r3

    d. 59 r2

35. 7050 − 305 =

    a. 6705

    b. 6745

    c. 5745

    d. 6045

36. 8327 − 1278 =

    a. 7149

    b. 7209

    c. 6059

    d. 7049

37. 285 × 12 =

    a. 3420

    b. 3402

    c. 3024

    d. 2322

38. 46 × 15 =

   a. 590

   b. 690

   c. 490

   d. 790

39. 5575 + 8791 =

   a. 14,756

   b. 14,566

   c. 14,466

   d. 14,366

40. What are the prime factors of 17?

   a. 2 x 8.5

   b. 17

   c. 3 x 5.5

   d. None of the above

41. What are the prime factors of 100?

   a. 2 x 2 x 5 x 5

   b. 4 x 25

   c. 2 x 2 x 2 x 5 x 5

   d. 2 x 50

Speed and Momentum

42. Three cars are travelling down an even road at a velocity of 110 m/s, calculate the car with the highest momentum if they are all moving at the same speed, but the first car weighs 2500 kg, second car weighs 2650 kg and third car weighs 2009 kg?

   a. First car

   b. Second car

   c. Third car

   d. All have same momentum

43. What is the momentum of a log of wood that weighs 700 kg rolling down a hill at 4.6 m/s?

   a. 3220 kg x m/s down hill

   b. 3320 kg x m/s

   c. 3320 down hill

   d. 3320 M

Quadratics and Polynomials

44. It is known that $x^2 + 4x = 5$. Then x can be

   a. 0

   b. -5

   c. 1

   d. Either (b) or (c)

45. Add $-3x^2 + 2x + 6$ and $-x^2 - x - 1$.

   a. $-2x^2 + x + 5$

   b. $-4x^2 + x + 5$

   c. $-2x^2 + 3x + 5$

   d. $-4x^2 + 3x + 5$

46. Simplify the following expression:

$3x^3 + 2x^2 + 5x - 7 + 4x^2 - 5x + 2 - 3x^3$

   a. $6x^2 - 9$

   b. $6x^2 - 5$

   c. $6x^2 - 10x - 5$

   d. $6x^2 + 10x - 9$

Scientific Notation

47. Convert 7,892,000,000 to scientific notation

    a. 7.892×10^{10}

    b. 7.892×10^{-9}

    c. 7.892×10^{9}

    d. 0.7892×10^{11}

48. Convert 0.045 to scientific notation

    a. 4.5×10^{-2}

    b. 4.5×10^{2}

    c. 4.05×10^{-2}

    d. 4.5×10^{-3}

Nonverbal IQ

Select the figure with the same relationship.

49.

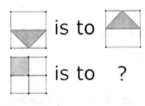

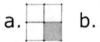

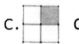

50.

Answer Key

Decimals, Percent and Fractions

1. D

With the new tax rate, income tax is 3.5%. Per month income tax = $9000/12 = $750. Per month income tax rate = $750 X 100/$25,000 = 3%. Income per month = $25,000 + $11,000 = $36,000. Monthly tax amount = $36,000 X 0.035 = $1260. Amount of addition tax = $1260 - $750 = $510

2. C

Total no. of balls = 10, no. of yellow balls = 2, answer = 2/10 X 100 = 20%

3. B

Suppose oranges in the basket before = x, Then: X + 8x/5 = 130, 5x + 8x = 650, so X = 50.

4. A

The area of a 7 centimeter pizza is $\prod(3.5)^2$ × = 38.48 cm². The weight of 1 cm² of pizza will be 750/38.48 = 19.49 grams. The area of 8.2 centimeter diameter pizza is $\prod (4.1)^2$ = 52.81 cm². The difference in area is 52.81 – 38.48 = 14.33 cm². The difference in weight will be 19.49 X 14.33 = 279.29 grams.

5. B

His distribution is: 300 kg - 20 × 15 - 6.4 × 15 = $96, 120 kg - 10 × 12 - 3.4 × 12 = $40.8, 130 kg - 5 × 26 - 1.8 × 26 = $46.8, Total = $183.6. Deducting the distribution cost, his net profit will be 183.6 – 175 = $13.60.

6. C

0.45 = 45/100 = 9/20

7. B

Let X be the total pay. X/2 – 250 = 3X/7, X = $3500.

8. B

$\sqrt{225}$ = 15.

9. B

(Amount Spent) $420 + $3000 (Balance) = $3420

10. B

9.60/3.2 = 3

11. A

20/100 = 45/X
X = 225

12. C

First convert to percent. 1/5 = 20%, so 10% of p = 20% of q, and p = 2 X q, and p - q = q

Basic Algebra

13. B

X = 7, so 3x = 3 x 7 = 21, 2x = 2 x 7 = 14, so 21 + 5 - 14 = 26 - 14 = 12

14. D

6x – 6 = 24 – 3x
6x + 3x - 6 = 24
9x – 6 = 24
9x = 24 + 6
9x = 30
x = 30/9
x = 3.33

15. A

Multiply the first bracket and the second. $x^2 - 3x + 7x - 21 = x^2 + 4x - 21$

Mean and Mode

16. B

First add all the numbers 100 + 1050 + 320 + 600 + 150 = 2220. Then divide by 5 (the number of data provided) = 2220/5 = 444

17. D

First arrange the numbers in a numerical sequence - 1,2,3,4,5,6,7,8,9, 10. Then find the middle number or numbers. The middle numbers are 5 and 6. The median = 5 + 6/2 = 11/2 = 5.5

18. B
Find the most recurring number. The most occurring number in the series is 9

Exponents

19. A
3 x 3 x 3 x 3 = 81

20. C
(4 x 4 x 4) + (2 x 2 x 2 x 2) = 64 + 16 = 80

21. D
$2(5)^3 - (2)^3 = 2(125) - 8 = 250 - 8 = 242$

22. D
$X^3 \times X^2 = X^{3+2} = X^5$
To multiply exponents with like bases, add the exponents.

23. A
Any value (except 0) raised to the power of 0 equals 1.

24. D
$\sqrt{144} = 12$

Geometry

25. B
The square with 2 cm side common to the rectangle apart from 4 cm side. So the perimeter = 2 + 2 + 2 + 4 + 2 + 4 = 16 cm.

26. C
Given: Two circles with a smaller circle (diameter given) exactly half the larger circle (radius given).
Difference = (Area of large circle) - (Area of small large circle)
$\pi 4^2 - \pi 2^2$
= 16π - 4π

Difference = 12π cm²

27. B
Pythagorean Theorem:
(Hypotenuse)^2 = (Perpendicular)^2 + (Base)^2
$h^2 = a^2 + b^2$

$a^2 = 81$, $b^2 = 144$
$h^2 = a^2 + b^2$
$h^2 = 81+144$
$h^2 = 225$
$h = 15$

28. C
The ratio of black balls to white is 38:42. Reduce to lowest terms = 19:21

29. D
The ratio 8:5 = X/100
X = 160%

30. D
First convert to inches – 4 X 12 = 48 sq. in. 48/3 = 16 sq. in.

31. B
In one round trip he covers the distance equal to the circumference of the circular path. 75/X = 3.14159. 75 X 3.14159 = X. Circumference of the path = X = 235.65 meters. Distance covered 7 times around = 235.65 × 7 = 1650 meters.

32. D
Indonesia is growing the fastest at about 30%.

33. A
467 × 41 = 19,147

34. B
1518 ÷ 27 = 56 r6

35. B
7050 – 305 = 6745

36. D
8327 – 1278 = 7049

37. A
285 × 12 = 3420

38. B
46 × 15 = 690

39. D
5575 + 8791 = 14366

40. B
The only prime number that can divide 17 is 17.

41. A
To make it easier we can break this large number to two smaller numbers, 2 x 50 or 4 x 25. Let's use 4 x 25. The prime factors of 4 = 2 x 2, and the prime factors of 25 = 5 x 5. The prime factors of 100 = 2 x 2 x 5 x 5

42. C
Momentum is a product of velocity and mass. If they are all travelling at the same speed, the car that weighs the most (the second car) would have the highest momentum.

43. A
The momentum of a log of wood that weighs 700kg rolling down a hill at 4.6m/s will be 4.6 X 700 = 3220 kg x m/s down hill.

Quadratics and Polynomials

44. D
$x^2 + 4x = 5$, $x^2 + 4x - 5 = 0$, $x^2 + 5x - x - 5 = 0$, factoring $x(x + 5) - 1(x + 5) = 0$, $(x + 5)(x-1)=0$. $x + 5 = 0$ or $x - 1 = 0$, $x = 0 - 5$ or $x = 0 + 1$, $x = -5$ or $x = 1$, either b or c.

45. B
$-4x^2 + x + 5$
$(-3x^2 + 2x + 6) + (-x^2 - x - 1)$
$-3x^2 + 2x + 6 - x^2 - x - 1$
$-4x^2 + x + 5$

46. B

$6x^2 - 5$

$3x^3 + 2x^2 + 5x - 7 + 4x^2 - 5x + 2 - 3x^3 = 6x^2 - 5$

Scientific Notation

47. C

The decimal point moves 9 spaces right to be placed after 7, which is the first non-zero number. Thus 7.892×10^9

48. A

The decimal point moves 2 spaces to the left to be placed before 4, which is the first non-zero number. Thus its 4.5×10^{-2} The answer is negative since the decimal moved left.

Nonverbal IQ

49. D

The relationship is the same figure flipped vertically, so the best choice is D.

50. C

The relation is the same figure with the bottom half removed.

Fraction Tips, Tricks and Shortcuts

When you are writing an exam, time is precious, and anything you can do to answer questions faster, is a real advantage. Here are some ideas, shortcuts, tips and tricks that can speed up answering fraction problems.

Remember that a fraction is just a number which names a portion of something. For instance, instead of having a whole pie, a fraction says you have a part of a pie--such as a half of one or a fourth of one.

Two digits make up a fraction. The digit on top is known as the numerator. The digit on the bottom is known as the denominator. To remember which is which, just remember that "denominator" and "down" both start with a "d." And the "downstairs" number is the denominator. So for instance, in ½, the numerator is the 1 and the denominator (or "downstairs") number is the 2.

- [ ] It's easy to add two fractions if they have the same denominator. Just add the digits on top and leave the bottom one the same: 1/10 + 6/10 = 7/10.

- [ ] It's the same with subtracting fractions with the same denominator: 7/10 - 6/10 = 1/10.

- [ ] Adding and subtracting fractions with different denominators is a little more complicated. First, you have to get the problem so that they do have the same denominators. One of the easiest ways to do this is to multiply the denominators: For 2/5 + 1/2 multiply 5 by 2. Now you have a denominator of 10. But now you have to change the top numbers too. Since you multiplied the 5 in 2/5 by 2, you also multiply the 2 by 2, to get 4. So the first number is now 4/10. Since you multiplied the second number times 5, you also multiply its top number by 5, to get a final fraction of 5/10. Now you can add 5 and 4 together to get a final sum of 9/10.

- [ ] Sometimes you'll be asked to reduce a fraction to its simplest form. This means getting it to where the only common factor of the numerator and denominator is 1. Think of it this way: Numerators and denominators are brothers that must be treated the same. If you do something to one, you must do it to the other, or it's just not fair. For instance, if you divide your numerator by 2, then you should also divide the denominator by the same. Let's take an example: The fraction 2/10 . This is not reduced to its simplest terms because there is a number that will divide evenly into both: the number 2. We want to make it so that the only number that will divide evenly into both is 1. What can we divide into 2 to get 1? The number 2, of course! Now to be "fair," we have to do the same thing to the denominator: Divide 2 into 10 and you get 5. So our new, reduced fraction is 1/5.

- [ ] In some ways, multiplying fractions is the easiest of all: Just multiply the two top numbers and then multiply the two bottom numbers. For instance, with this problem:
  2/5 X 2/3 you multiply 2 by 2 and get a top number of 4; then multiply 5 by 3 and get a bottom number of 15. Your answer is 4/15.

☐   Dividing fractions is a bit more involved, but still not too hard. You once again multiply, but only AFTER you have turned the second fraction upside-down. To divide ⅞ by ½, turn the ½ into 2/1, then multiply the top numbers and multiply the bottom numbers: ⅞ X 2/1 gives us 14 on top and 8 on the bottom.

Converting Fractions to Decimals

There are a couple of ways to become good at converting fractions to decimals. One -- the one that will make you the fastest in basic math skills -- is to learn some basic fraction facts. It's a good idea, if you're good at memory, to memorize the following:

1/100 is "one hundredth," expressed as a decimal, it's .01.

1/50 is "two hundredths," expressed as a decimal, it's .02.

1/25 is "one twenty-fifths" or "four hundredths," expressed as a decimal, it's .04.

1/20 is "one twentieth" or ""five hundredths," expressed as a decimal, it's .05.

1/10 is "one tenth," expressed as a decimal, it's .1.

1/8 is "one eighth," or "one hundred twenty-five thousandths," expressed as a decimal, it's .125.

1/5 is "one fifth," or "two tenths," expressed as a decimal, it's .2.

1/4 is "one fourth" or "twenty-five hundredths," expressed as a decimal, it's .25.

1/3 is "one third" or "thirty-three hundredths," expressed as a decimal, it's .33.

1/2 is "one half" or "five tenths," expressed as a decimal, it's .5.

3/4 is "three fourths," or "seventy-five hundredths," expressed as a decimal, it's .75.

Of course, if you're no good at memorization, another good technique for converting a fraction to a decimal is to manipulate it so that the fraction's denominator is 10, 10, 1000, or some other power of 10. Here's an example: We'll start with ¾. What is the first number in the 4 "times table" that you can multiply and get a multiple of 10? Can you multiply 4 by something to get 10? No. Can you multiply it by something to get 100? Yes! 4 X 25 is 100. So let's take that 25 and multiply it by the numerator in our fraction ¾. The numerator is 3, and 3 X 25 is 75. We'll move the decimal in 75 all the way to the left, and we find that ¾ is .75.

We'll do another one: 1/5. Again, we want to find a power of 10 that 5 goes into evenly. Will 5 go into 10? Yes! It goes 2 times. So we'll take that 2 and multiply it by our numerator, 1, and we get 2. We move the decimal in 2 all the way to the left and find that 1/5 is equal to .2.

Converting Fractions to Percent

Working with either fractions or percents can be intimidating enough. But converting from one to the other? That's a genuine nightmare for those who are not math wizards. But really, it doesn't have to be that way. Here are two ways to make it easier and faster to convert a fraction to a percent.

☐ First, you might remember that a fraction is nothing more than a division problem: you're dividing the bottom number into the top number. So for instance, if we start with a fraction 1/10, we are making a division problem with the 10 on the outside of the bracket and the 1 on the inside. As you remember from your lessons on dividing by decimals, since 10 won't go into 1, you add a decimal and make it 10 into 1.0. 10 into 10 goes 1 time, and since it's behind the decimal, it's .1. And how do we say .1? We say "one tenth," which is exactly what we started with: 1/10. So we have a number we can work with now: .1. When we're dealing with percents, though, we're dealing strictly with hundredths (not tenths). You remember from studying decimals that adding a zero to the right of the number on the right side of the decimal does not change the value. Therefore, we can change .1 into .10 and have the same number--except now it's expressed as hundredths. We have 10 hundredths. That's ten out of 100--which is just another way of saying ten percent (ten per hundred or ten out of 100). In other words .1 = .10 = 10 percent. Remember, if you're changing from a decimal to a percent, get rid of the decimal on the left and replace it with a percent mark on the right: 10%. Let's review those steps again: Divide 10 into 1. Since 10 doesn't go into 1, turn 1 into 1.0. Now divide 10 into 1.0. Since 10 goes into 10 1 time, put it there and add your decimal to make it .1. Since a percent is always "hundredths," let's change .1 into .10. Then remove the decimal on the left and replace with a percent sign on the right. The answer is 10%.

☐ If you're doing these conversions on a multiple-choice test, here's an idea that might be even easier and faster. Let's say you have a fraction of 1/8 and you're asked what the percent is. Since we know that "percent" means hundredths, ask yourself what number we can multiply 8 by to get 100. Since there is no number, ask what number gets us close to 100. That number is 12: 8 X 12 = 96. So it gets us a little less than 100. Now, whatever you do to the denominator, you have to do to the numerator. Let's multiply 1 X 12 and we get 12. However, since 96 is a little less than 100, we know that our answer will be a percent a little MORE than 12%. So if your possible answers on the multiple-choice test are these:

a) 8.5%   b) 19%   c)12.5%   d) 25%

then we know the answer is c) 12.5%, because it's a little MORE than the 12 we got in our math problem above.

Another way to look at this, using multiple choice strategy is you know the answer will be "about" 12. Looking at the other choices, they are all either too large or too small and can be eliminated right away.

This was an easy example to demonstrate, so don't be fooled! You probably won't get such an easy question on your exam, but the principle holds just the same. By estimating your answer quickly, you can eliminate choices immediately and save precious exam time.

Decimal Tips, Tricks and Shortcuts

Converting Decimals to Fractions

One of the most important tricks for correctly converting a decimal to a fraction doesn't involve math at all. It's simply to learn to say the decimal correctly. If you say "point one" or "point 25" for .1 and .25, you'll have more trouble getting the conversion correct. But if you know that it's called "one tenth" and "twenty-five hundredths," you're on the way to a correct conversion. That's because, if you know your fractions, you know that "one tenth" looks like this: 1/10. And "twenty-five hundredths" looks like this: 25/100.

Even if you have digits before the decimal, such as 3.4, learning how to say the word will help you with the conversion into a fraction. It's not "three point four," it's "three and four tenths." Knowing this, you know that the fraction which looks like "three and four tenths" is 3 4/10.

Of course, your conversion is not complete until you reduce the fraction to its lowest terms: It's not 25/100, but 1/4.

Converting Decimals to Percent

Changing a decimal to a percent is easy if you remember one math formula: multiply by 100. For instance, if you start with .45, you change it to a percent by simply multiplying it by 100. You then wind up with 45. Add the % sign to the end and you get 45%.

That seems easy enough, right? In this case think of it this way: You just take out the decimal and stick in a percent sign on the opposite sign. In other words, the decimal on the left is replaced by the % on the right.

It doesn't work quite that easily if the decimal is in the middle of the number. Let's use 3.7 as an example. In this case, take out the decimal in the middle and replace it with a 0 % at the end. So 3.7 converted to decimal is 370%.

Percent Tips, Tricks and Shortcuts

Percent problems are not nearly as scary as they appear, if you remember this neat trick:

Draw a cross as in:

Portion	Percent
Whole	100

In the upper left, write PORTION. In the bottom left write WHOLE. In the top right, write PERCENT and in the bottom right, write 100. Whatever your problem is, you will leave blank the unknown, and fill in the other four parts. For example, let's suppose your problem is: Find 10% of 50. Since we know the 10% part, we put 10 in the percent corner. Since the whole number in our problem is 50, we put that in the corner marked whole. You always put 100 underneath the percent, so we leave it as is, which leaves only the top left corner blank. This is where we'll put our answer. Now simply multiply the two corner numbers that are NOT 100. In this case, it's 10 X 50. That gives us 500. Now multiply this by the remaining corner, or 100, to get a final answer of 5. 5 is the number that goes in the upper-left corner, and is your final solution.

Another hint to remember: Percents are the same thing as hundredths in decimals. So .45 is the same as 45 hundredths or 45 percent.

Converting Percents to Decimals

Percents are simply a specific type of decimals, so it should be no surprise that converting between the two is actually fairly simple. Here are a few tricks and shortcuts to keep in mind:

- ☐ Remember that percent literally means "per 100" or "for every 100." So when you speak of 30% you're saying 30 for every 100 or the fraction 30/100. In basic math, you learned that fractions that have 10 or 100 as the denominator can easily be turned into a decimal. 30/100 is thirty hundredths, or expressed as a decimal, .30.
- ☐ Another way to look at it: To convert a percent to a decimal, simply divide the number by 100. So for instance, if the percent is 47%, divide 47 by 100. The result will be .47. Get rid of the % mark and you're done.
- ☐ Remember that the easiest way of dividing by 100 is by moving your decimal two spots to the left.

Converting Percents to Fractions

Converting percents to fractions is easy. After all, a percent is nothing except a type of fraction; it tells you what part of 100 that you're talking about. Here are some simple ideas for making the conversion from a percent to a fraction:

- ☐ If the percent is a whole number -- say 34% -- then simply write a fraction with 100 as the denominator (the bottom number). Then put the percentage itself on top. So 34% becomes 34/100.

☐ Now reduce as you would reduce any percent. In this case, by dividing 2 into 34 and 2 into 100, you get 17/50.

☐ If your percent is not a whole number -- say 3.4% --then convert it to a decimal expressed as hundredths. 3.4 is the same as 3.40 (or 3 and forty hundredths). Now ask yourself how you would express "three and forty hundredths" as a fraction. It would, of course, be 3 40/100. Reduce this and it becomes 3 2/5.

How to Answer Basic Math Multiple Choice

Math is the one section where you need to make sure that you understand the processes before you ever tackle it. That's because the time allowed on the math portion is typically so short that there's not much room for error. You have to be fast and accurate. It's imperative that before the test day arrives, you've learned all of the main formulas that will be used, and then to create your own problems (and solve them).

On the actual test day, use the "Plug-Check-Check" strategy. Here's how it goes.

Read the problem, but not the answers. You'll want to work the problem first and come up with your own answers. If you did the work right, you should find your answer among the options given.

If you need help with the problem, plug actual numbers into the variables given. You'll find it easier to work with numbers than it is to work with letters. For instance, if the question asks, "If Y-4 is 2 more than Z, then Y+5 is how much more than Z?" try selecting a value for Y. Let's take 6. Your question now becomes, "If 6-4 is 2 more than Z, then 6 plus 5 is how much more than Z?" Now your answer should be easier to work with.

Check the answer options to see if your answer matches one of those. If so, select it.

If no answer matches the one you got, re-check your math, but this time, use a different method. In math, it's common for there to be more than one way to solve a problem. As a simple example, if you multiplied 12 X 13 and did not get an answer that matches one of the answer options, you might try adding 13 together 12 different times and see if you get a good answer.

Math Multiple Choice Strategy

The two strategies for working with basic math multiple choice are Estimation and Elimination.

Math Strategy 1 - Estimation.

Just like it sounds, try to estimate an approximate answer first. Then look at the choices.

Math Strategy 2 - Elimination.

For every question, no matter what type, eliminating obviously incorrect answers narrows the possible choices. Elimination is probably the most powerful strategy for answering multiple choice.

Here are a few basic math examples of how this works.

Solve 2/3 + 5/12

     a. 9/17

     b. 3/11

     c. 7/12

     d. 1 1/12

First estimate the answer. 2/3 is more than half and 5/12 is about half, so the answer is going to be very close to 1.

Next, Eliminate. Choice A is about 1/2 and can be eliminated, Choice B is very small, less than 1/2 and can be eliminated. Choice C is close to 1/2 and can be eliminated. Leaving only Choice D, which is just over 1.

Work through the solution, a common denominator is needed, a number which both 3 and 12 will divide into.
2/3 = 8/12. So, 8+5/12 = 13/12 = 1 1/12

Choice D is correct.

Solve 4/5 – 2/3

     a. 2/2

     b. 2/13

     c. 1

     d. 2/15

You can eliminate Choice A, because it is 1 and since both of the numbers are close to one, the difference is going to be very small. You can eliminate Choice C for the same reason.

Next, look at the denominators. Since 5 and 3 don't go in to 13, you can eliminate Choice B as well.

That leaves Choice D.

Checking the answer, the common denominator will be 15. So 12-10/15 = 2/15. Choice D is correct.

Fractions shortcut - Cancelling out.

In any operation with fractions, if the numerator of one fractions has a common multiple with the denominator of the other, you can cancel out. This saves time and simplifies the problem quickly, making it easier to manage.

Solve 2/15 ÷ 4/5

> a. 6/65
> b. 6/75
> c. 5/12
> d. 1/6

To divide fractions, we multiply the first fraction with the inverse of the second fraction. Therefore we have
2/15 x 5/4. The numerator of the first fraction, 2, shares a multiple with the denominator of the second fraction, 4, which is 2. These cancel out, which gives, 1/3 x 1/2 = 1/6

Cancelling Out solved the questions very quickly, but we can still use multiple choice strategies to answer.

Choice B can be eliminated because 75 is too large a denominator. Choice C can be eliminated because 5 and 15 don't go in to 12.

Choice D is correct.

Decimal Multiple Choice strategy and Shortcuts.

Multiplying decimals gives a very quick way to estimate and eliminate choices. Anytime that you multiply decimals, it is going to give a answer with the same number of decimal places as the combined operands.

So for example,

2.38 X 1.2 will produce a number with three places of decimal, which is 2.856.

Here are a few examples with step-by-step explanation:

Solve 2.06 x 1.2

    a. 24.82

    b. 2.482

    c. 24.72

    d. 2.472

This is a simple question, but even before you start calculating, you can eliminate several choices. When multiplying decimals, there will always be as many numbers behind the decimal place in the answer as the sum of the ones in the initial problem, so Choice A and C can be eliminate.

The correct answer is D: 2.06 x 1.2 = 2.472

Solve 20.0 ÷ 2.5

    a. 12.05

    b. 9.25

    c. 8.3

    d. 8

First estimate the answer to be around 10, and eliminate Choice A. And since it'd also be an even number, you can eliminate Choice B and C., leaving only choice D.

The correct Answer is D: 20.0 ÷ 2.5 = 8

How to Solve Word Problems

Most students find math word problems difficult. Tackling word problems is much easier if you have a systematic approach which we outline below.

Here is the biggest tip for studying word problems.

Practice regularly and systematically. Sounds simple and easy right? Yes it is, and yes it really does work.

Word problems are a way of thinking and require you to translate a real word problem into mathematical terms.

Some math instructors go so far as to say that learning how to think mathematically is the main reason for teaching word problems.

So what do we mean by Practice regularly and systematically? Studying word problems and math in general requires a logical and mathematical frame of mind. The only way you can get this is by practicing regularly, which means everyday.

It is critical that you practice word problems everyday for the 5 days before the exam as a bare minimum.

If you practice and miss a day, you have lost the mathematical frame of mind and the benefit of your previous practice is pretty much gone. Anyone who has done any amount of math will agree – you have to practice everyday.

Everything is important. The other critical point about word problems is that all of the information given in the problem has some purpose. There is no unnecessary information! Word problems are typically around 50 words in 1 to 3 sentences. If the sometimes complicated relationships are to be explained in that short an explanation, every word has to count. Make sure that you use every piece of information.

Here are 9 simple steps to help you resolve word problems.

Step 1 – Read through the problem at least three times. The first reading should be a quick scan, and the next two readings should be done slowly with a view to finding answers to these important questions:

What does the problem ask? (Usually located towards the end of the problem)

What does the problem imply? (This is usually a point you were asked to remember).

Mark all information, and underline all important words or phrases.

Step 2 – Try to make a pictorial representation of the problem such as a circle and an arrow to indicate travel. This makes the problem a bit more real and sensible to you.

A favorite word problem is something like, 1 train leaves Station A travelling at 100 km/hr and another train leaves Station B travelling at 60 km/hr. ...

Draw a line, the two stations, and the two trains at either end. This will help solidify the situation in your mind.

Step 3 – Use the information you have to make a table with a blank portion to indicate information you do not know.

Step 4 – Assign a single letter to represent each unknown data in your table. You can write down the unknown that each letter represents so that you do not make the error of assigning answers to the wrong unknown, because a word problem may have multiple unknowns and you will need to create equations for each unknown.

Step 5 – Translate the English terms in the word problem into a mathematical algebraic equation. Remember that the main problem with word problems is that they are not expressed in regular math equations. You ability to correctly identify the variables and translate the word problem into an equation determines your ability to solve the problem.

Step 6 – Check the equation to see if it looks like regular equations that you are used to seeing and whether it looks sensible. Does the equation appear to represent the information in the question? Take note that you may need to rewrite some formulas needed to solve the word problem equation. For example, word distance problems may need you rewriting the distance formula, which is Distance = Time x Rate. If the word problem requires that you solve for time you will need to use Distance/Rate and Distance/Time to solve for Rate. If you understand the distance word problem you should be able to identify the variable you need to solve for.

Step 7 – Use algebra rules to solve the derived equation. Take note that the laws of equation demands that what is done on this side of the equation has to also be done on the other side. You have to solve the equation so that the unknown ends up alone on one side. Where there are multiple unknowns you will need to use elimination or substitution methods to resolve all the equations.

Step 8 – Check your final answers to see if they make sense with the information given in the problem. For example if the word problem involves a discount, the final price should be less or if a product was taxed then the final answer has to cost more.

Step 9 – Cross check your answers by placing the answer or answers in the first equation to replace the unknown or unknowns. If your answer is correct then both side of the equation must equate or equal. If your answer is not correct then you may have derived a wrong equation or solved the equation wrongly. Repeat the necessary steps to correct.

Types of Word Problems

Word problems can be classified into 12 types. Below are examples of each type with a complete solution. Some types of word problems can be solved quickly using multiple choice strategies and some can not. Always look for ways to estimate the answer and then eliminate choices.

1. Age

A girl is 10 years older than her brother. By next year, she will be twice the age of her brother. What are their ages now?

    a. 25, 15
    b. 19, 9
    c. 21, 11
    d. 29, 19

Solution: B

We will assume that the girl's age is "a" and her brother's is "b". This means that based

on the information in the first sentence,
a = 10 + b

Next year, she will be twice her brother's age, which gives
a + 1 = 2(b+1)

We need to solve for one unknown factor and then use the answer to solve for the other. To do this we substitute the value of "a" from the first equation into the second equation. This gives
10+b + 1 = 2b + 2
11 + b = 2b + 2
11 – 2 = 2b – b
b= 9

9 = b this means that her brother is 9 years old. Solving for the girl's age in the first equation gives a = 10 + 9. a = 19 the girl is aged 19. So, the girl is aged 19 and the boy is 9

2. Distance or speed

Two boats travel down a river towards the same destination, starting at the same time. One of the boats is traveling at 52 km/hr, and the other boat at 43 km/hr. How far apart will they be after 40 minutes?

     a. 46.67 km

     b. 19.23 km

     c. 6.4 km

     d. 14.39 km

Solution: C

After 40 minutes, the first boat will have traveled = 52 km/hr x 40 minutes/60 minutes = 34.7 km
After 40 minutes, the second boat will have traveled = 43 km/hr x 40/60 minutes = 28.66 km
Difference between the two boats will be 34.7 km – 28.66 km = 6.04 km.

Multiple Choice Strategy

First estimate the answer. The first boat is travelling 9 km. faster than the second, for 40 minutes, which is 2/3 of an hour. 2/3 of 9 = 6, as a rough guess of the distance apart.

Choices A, B and D can be eliminated right away.

3. Ratio

The instructions in a cookbook states that 700 grams of flour must be mixed in 100 ml of water, and 0.90 grams of salt added. A cook however has just 325 grams of flour. What is the quantity of water and salt that he should use?

    a. 0.41 grams and 46.4 ml

    b. 0.45 grams and 49.3 ml

    c. 0.39 grams and 39.8 ml

    d. 0.25 grams and 40.1 ml

Solution: A

The Cookbook states 700 grams of flour, but the cook only has 325. The first step is to determine the percentage of flour he has 325/700 x 100 = 46.4%
That means that 46.4% of all other items must also be used.
46.4% of 100 = 46.4 ml of water
46.4% of 0.90 = 0.41 grams of salt.

Multiple Choice Strategy

The recipe calls for 700 grams of flour but the cook only has 325, which is just less than half, the amount of water and salt are going to be approximately half.

Choices C and D can be eliminated right away. Choice B is very close so be careful. Looking closely at Choice B, it is exactly half, and since 325 is slightly less than half of 700, it can't be correct.

Choice A is correct.

4. Percent

An agent received $6,685 as his commission for selling a property. If his commission was 13% of the selling price, how much was the property?

    a. $68,825

    b. $121,850

    c. $49,025

    d. $51,423

Solution: D

Let's assume that the property price is x
That means from the information given, 13% of x = 6,685
Solve for x,
x = 6685 x 100/13 = $51,423

Multiple Choice Strategy

The commission,13%, is just over 10%, which is easier to work with. Round up $6685 to $6700, and multiple by 10 for an approximate answer. 10 X 6700 = $67,000. You can do this in your head. Choice B is much too big and can be eliminated. Choice C is too small and can be eliminated. Choices A and D are left and good possibilities.

Do the calculations to make the final choice.

5. Sales & Profit

A store owner buys merchandise for $21,045. He transports them for $3,905 and pays his staff $1,450 to stock the merchandise on his shelves. If he does not incur further costs, how much does he need to sell the items to make $5,000 profit?

  a. $32,500
  b. $29,350
  c. $32,400
  d. $31,400

Solution: D

Total cost of the items is $21,045 + $3,905 + $1,450 = $26,400
Total cost is now $26,400 + $5000 profit = $31,400

Multiple Choice Strategy

Round off and add the numbers up in your head quickly.
21,000 + 4,000 + 1500 = 26500. Add in 5000 profit for a total of 31500.

Choice B is too small and can be eliminated. Choice C and Choice A are too large and can be eliminated.

6. Tax/Income

A woman earns $42,000 per month and pays 5% tax on her monthly income. If the Government increases her monthly taxes by $1,500, what is her income after tax?

  a. $38,400
  b. $36,050
  c. $40,500
  d. $39, 500

Solution: A

Initial tax on income was 5/100 x 42,000 = $2,100
$1,500 was added to the tax to give $2,100 + 1,500 = $3,600
Income after tax left is $42,000 - $3,600 = $38,400

7. Interest

A man invests $3000 in a 2-year term deposit that pays 3% interest per year. How much will he have at the end of the 2-year term?

    a. $5,200
    b. $3,020
    c. $3,182.7
    d. $3,000

Solution: C

This is a compound interest problem. The funds are invested for 2 years and interest is paid yearly, so in the second year, he will earn interest on the interest paid in the first year.

3% interest in the first year = 3/100 x 3,000 = $90
At end of first year, total amount = 3,000 + 90 = $3,090
Second year = 3/100 x 3,090 = 92.7.
At end of second year, total amount = $3090 + $92.7 = $3,182.7

8. Averaging

The average weight of 10 books is 54 grams. 2 more books were added and the average weight became 55.4. If one of the 2 new books added weighed 62.8 g, what is the weight of the other?

    a. 44.7 g
    b. 67.4 g
    c. 62 g
    d. 52 g

Solution: C
Total weight of 10 books with average 54 grams will be=10×54=540 g
Total weight of 12 books with average 55.4 will be=55.4×12=664.8 g
So total weight of the remaining 2 will be= 664.8 – 540 = 124.8 g
If one weighs 62.8, the weight of the other will be= 124.8 g – 62.8 g = 62 g

Multiple Choice Strategy

Averaging problems can be estimated by looking at which direction the average goes. If additional items are added and the average goes up, the new items much be greater than the average. If the average goes down after new items are added, the new items must be less than the average.

In this case, the average is 54 grams and 2 books are added which increases the average to 55.4, so the new books must weight more than 54 grams.

Choices A and D can be eliminated right away.

9. Probability

A bag contains 15 marbles of various colors. If 3 marbles are white, 5 are red and the rest are black, what is the probability of randomly picking out a black marble from the bag?

    a. 7/15
    b. 3/15
    c. 1/5
    d. 4/15

Solution: A

Total marbles = 15
Number of black marbles = 15 – (3 + 5) = 7
Probability of picking out a black marble = 7/15

10. Two Variables

A company paid a total of $2850 to book for 6 single rooms and 4 double rooms in a hotel for one night. Another company paid $3185 to book for 13 single rooms for one night in the same hotel. What is the cost for single and double rooms in that hotel?

    a. single= $250 and double = $345
    b. single= $254 and double = $350
    c. single = $245 and double = $305
    d. single = $245 and double = $345

Solution: D

We can determine the price of single rooms from the information given of the second company. 13 single rooms = 3185.
One single room = 3185 / 13 = 245
The first company paid for 6 single rooms at $245. 245 x 6 = $1470
Total amount paid for 4 double rooms by first company = $2850 - $1470 = $1380
Cost per double room = 1380 / 4 = $345

11. Geometry

The length of a rectangle is 5 in. more than its width. The perimeter of the rectangle is 26 in. What is the width and length of the rectangle?

   a. width = 6 inches, Length = 9 inches
   b. width = 4 inches, Length = 9 inches
   c. width = 4 inches, Length = 5 inches
   d. width = 6 inches, Length = 11 inches

Solution: B

Formula for perimeter of a rectangle is 2(L + W)
p=26, so 2(L+W) = p
The length is 5 inches more than the width, so
2(w+5) + 2w = 26
2w + 10 + 2w = 26
2w + 2w = 26 - 10
4w = 18

W = 16/4 = 4 inches

L is 5 inches more than w, so L = 5 + 4 = 9 inches.

12. Totals and fractions

A basket contains 125 oranges, mangos and apples. If 3/5 of the fruits in the basket are mangos and only 2/5 of the mangos are ripe, how many ripe mangos are there in the basket?

   a. 30
   b. 68
   c. 55
   d. 47

Solution: A
Number of mangos in the basket is 3/5 x 125 = 75
Number of ripe mangos = 2/5 x 75 = 30

Exponents: Tips, Shortcuts & Tricks

Exponents seem like advanced math to most—like some mysterious code with a complicated meaning. In fact, though, an exponent is just short hand for saying that you're multiplying a number by itself two or more times. For instance, instead of saying that you're multiplying 5 x 5 x 5, you can show that you're multiplying 5 by itself 3 times if you just write 53 .We usually say this as "five to the third power" or "five to the power of three." In this example, the raised 3 is an "exponent," while the 5 is the "base." You can even use exponents with fractions. For instance, ½ 3 means you're multiplying ½ x ½ x ½. (The answer is 1/8). Some other helpful hints for working with exponents:

•   Here's how to do basic multiplication of exponents. If you have the same number with a different exponent (For instance 53 X 52) just add the exponents and multiply the bases as usual. The answer, then, is 255 .

•   This doesn't work, though, if the bases are different. For instance, in 53 X 32
we simply have to do the math the long way to figure out the final solution: 5 x 5 x 5,   multiplying that result times the result for 3 X 2. (The answer is 750).

•   Looking at it from the opposite side, to divide two exponents with the same base (or bottom number), subtract the smaller exponent from the larger one. If we were dividing the problem above, we would subtract the 2 from the 3 to get 1. 5 to the power of 1 is simply 5.

•   One time when thinking of exponents as merely multiplication doesn't work is when the raised number is zero. Any number raised to the "zeroth" power is 1 (Not, as we tend to think, zero).

Number (x)	X^2	X^3
1	1	1
2	4	8
3	9	27
4	16	64
5	25	125
6	36	216
7	49	343
8	64	512
9	81	729
10	100	1000

Mean, Median and Mode

Mean, mode and median are basic statistical tools used to calculate different types of averages.

Mean

Mean is the most common form of average used. To calculate mean, you simple add up all the values of data given and divide by the number data provided.

Example

Find the mean of 8, 5, 7, 10, 15, 21
Sum of values = 8 + 5 + 7 + 10 + 15 + 21 = 66
Number of data = 6
Mean = 66/6 = 11

Median

Median refers to the middle value among a set or series of values after they have been arranged in numerical order. Median thus means the middle of the set of values. When two numbers fall in the middle, you simple add the value of the two numbers and divide by 2 to get the middle of the two numbers.

Example

Arrange these numbers in ascending order and then find the median

First arrange in ascending order 8, 5, 7, 10, 15, 21
= 5, 7, 8, 10, 15, 21

There are 6 numbers on the series and two fall in the middle = 8 and 10
The median = 8 + 10/2
= 18/2 = 9

Mode

Mode refers to the most occurring number or value among a set of values. It is important to note that it is possible not to have a most occurring number and then the answer becomes 'No Mode'

Example

8, 5, 7, 10, 15, 21, 5, 7, 2, 5

Mode refers to the most occurring number

8, 10, 15, 2 and 21 occur once
5 occurs 3 times
7 occurs 2 times

The most occurring number is 5, which occurs three times.

Order Of Operation

Some math calculations contain more than one set of operations. For example, a problem like 3 + (35 - 21) x 2 requires addition, subtraction and multiplication operations. The problem arises from the confusion of which of the operations to perform first. Starting with the wrong operation will give you the wrong answer. To solve this dilemma and to avoid confusion, the Order of Operation rules were set.

Order of operation is a set of mathematical rules designed to be used for calculations that require more than one arithmetic operation. For example, calculation problems that require two or more out of addition, subtraction, multiplication and division, would require that you follow the order of operation to solve.

The order of operation rules are quite simple as explained below.

Rule 1: Start with calculations that are inside brackets or parentheses.
Rule 2: Then, solve all multiplications and divisions, from left to right.
Rule 3: Finally, solve all additions and subtractions, from left to right.

Example 1

Solve 16 + 5 x 8

Based on the rules above, we would have to start with the multiplication part of the question.
That will give: 16 + 40 = 56

Take note that if the rule was not followed and addition was done first, the answer gotten would be different and wrong.

16 + 5 x 8
21 x 8 = 168 (wrong answer)

Example 2

3 +(35 - 21) x 2

Based on the rules of the order of operation, we have to solve the problem in the bracket or parenthesis first. Then we do the multiplication, before doing the addition.

3 + (35 - 21) x 2
3 + (14) x 3
3 + 42
= 45

Scientific Notation

Scientific notation is a very simple and effective way of representing very large numbers in simpler forms. For example, instead of writing out 149,600,000,000 meters, which is the estimated distance from the sun, astronomers could easily write it out as 1.496×10^{11} meters

Scientific notation expresses numbers in their powers of ten. It can be used to even express simple numbers.

For example, using scientific notation, $10 = 10^1$ The exponent "1" tells the number of times to multiply by 10 to get the original number.

$100 = 10^2$

$1000 = 10^3$

$10^0 = 1$

When the exponent is negative, it tells us how many times we need to divide by ten to get the original number.

For example, $0.025 = 2.5 \times 10$

The accepted format of scientific notation or writing numbers on their powers of 10 is a $\times 10^n$

Where a must be between 1 and 10 and n must be an integer

How to convert to scientific notation

To convert a number to scientific notation, you would need to place a decimal after the first number that is not a zero or after the first number that ranges between 1 and 9.

After placing the decimal, you need to count the number of places that the decimal had to move to get the exponent of 10. If the decimal moves to the left, then the exponent to multiply 10 will be in the positive. If the decimal moves from right to left, we will then have a negative power of 10.

For example, to convert 29010, we need to place a decimal after 2, since 2 is the first non zero number. We would then have 2.91

If we were to convert 0.0167, we need to place the decimal after 1, since the first two numbers before 1 were zeros and do not fall between 1 and 9. We would thus have 1.67

To complete the conversion of 29010 to scientific notation, we would get 2.91×10^4

The 10 is raised to the power of 4, because there are 4 places counting from the right to left where the decimal had to move. This scientific notation is in the positive because the decimal moved to the left.

$0.0167 = 1.67 \times 10^{-2}$

In this example, the decimal place moved from left to right by 2 spaces thus the 10 is raised to the power of 2. It is in the negative, because the decimal moved towards the right.

How to convert from scientific notation

You may also need to convert numbers that are already represented in scientific notation or in their power of ten to regular numbers. It is quite easy.

First it is important to remember these two laws.

If the power is in the positive, shift decimal to the right
If the power is in the negative, shift decimal point to the left

Example

Convert 3.201×10^3

This scientific notation is in the positive so we just need to shift the decimal to the right by 2 spaces, which is the power of the 10. We thus have: $3.201 \times 10^3 = 3201$

Another example

Convert

1.03×10^{-4}

The scientific notation here is negative and so we need to shift decimal to the left. Thus $1.03 \times 10^{-2} = 0.000103$ The decimal was shifted 4 spaces to the left.

Ratios

In mathematics, a ratio is a relationship between two numbers of the same kind[1] (e.g., objects, persons, students, spoonfuls, units of whatever identical dimension), usually expressed as "a to b" or a:b, sometimes expressed arithmetically as a dimensionless quotient of the two[2] which explicitly indicates how many times the first number contains the second (not necessarily an integer).[3] In layman's terms a ratio represents, simply, for every amount of one thing, how much there is of another thing. For example, suppose I have 10 pairs of socks for every pair of shoes then the ratio of shoes:socks would be 1:10 and the ratio of socks:shoes would be 10:1.

Notation and terminology

The ratio of numbers A and B can be expressed as:[4]
the ratio of A to B
A is to B
A:B

A rational number which is the quotient of A divided by B
The numbers A and B are sometimes called terms with A being the antecedent and B being the consequent.

The proportion expressing the equality of the ratios A:B and C:D is written A:B=C:D or A:B::C:D. this latter form, when spoken or written in the English language, is often expressed as
A is to B as C is to D.

Again, A, B, C, D are called the terms of the proportion. A and D are called the extremes, and B and C are called the means. The equality of three or more proportions is called a continued proportion.[5]
Ratios are sometimes used with three or more terms. The dimensions of a two by four that is ten inches long are 2:4:10.

Examples

The quantities being compared in a ratio might be physical quantities such as speed or length, or numbers of objects, or amounts of particular substances. A common example of the last case is the weight ratio of water to cement used in concrete, which is commonly stated as 1:4. This means that the weight of cement used is four times the weight of water used. It does not say anything about the total amounts of cement and water used, nor the amount of concrete being made. Equivalently it could be said that the ratio of cement to water is 4:1, that there is 4 times as much cement as water, or that there is a quarter (1/4) as much water as cement..
Older televisions have a 4:3 "aspect ratio", which means that the width is 4/3 of the height; modern widescreen TVs have a 16:9 aspect ratio.

Fractional

If there are 2 oranges and 3 apples, the ratio of oranges to apples is 2:3, and the ratio of oranges to the total number of pieces of fruit is 2:5. These ratios can also be expressed in fraction form: there are 2/3 as many oranges as apples, and 2/5 of the pieces of fruit are oranges. If orange juice concentrate is to be diluted with water in the ratio 1:4, then one part of concentrate is mixed with four parts of water, giving five parts total; the amount of orange juice concentrate is 1/4 the amount of water, while the amount of orange juice concentrate is 1/5 of the total liquid. In both ratios and fractions, it is important to be clear what is being compared to what, and beginners often make mistakes for this reason.

Number of terms

In general, when comparing the quantities of a two-quantity ratio, this can be expressed as a fraction derived from the ratio. For example, in a ratio of 2:3, the amount/size/volume/number of the first quantity will be that of the second quantity. This pattern also works with ratios with more than two terms. However, a ratio with more than two terms cannot be completely converted into a single fraction; a single fraction represents only one part of the ratio since a fraction can only compare two numbers. If the ratio deals with objects or amounts of objects, this is often expressed as "for every two parts of the first quantity there are three parts of the second quantity".

Percent and ratio

If we multiply all quantities involved in a ratio by the same number, the ratio remains valid. For example, a ratio of 3:2 is the same as 12:8. It is usual either to reduce terms to the lowest common denominator, or to express them in parts per hundred (percent).

If a mixture contains substances A, B, C & D in the ratio 5:9:4:2 then there are 5 parts of A for every 9 parts of B, 4 parts of C and 2 parts of D. As 5+9+4+2=20, the total mixture contains 5/20 of A (5 parts out of 20), 9/20 of B, 4/20 of C, and 2/20 of D. If we divide all numbers by the total and multiply by 100, this is converted to percentages: 25% A, 45% B, 20% C, and 10% D (equivalent to writing the ratio as 25:45:20:10).

Proportion

If the two or more ratio quantities encompass all of the quantities in a particular situation, for example two apples and three oranges in a fruit basket containing no other types of fruit, it could be said that "the whole" contains five parts, made up of two parts apples and three parts oranges. In this case, or 40% of the whole are apples or 60% of the whole are oranges. This comparison of a specific quantity to "the whole" is sometimes called a proportion. Proportions are sometimes expressed as percentages as demonstrated above.

Reduction

Note that ratios can be reduced (as fractions are) by dividing each quantity by the common factors of all the quantities. This is often called "cancelling." As for fractions, the simplest form is considered to be that in which the numbers in the ratio are the smallest possible integers.

Thus, the ratio 40:60 may be considered equivalent in meaning to the ratio 2:3 within contexts concerned only with relative quantities.

Mathematically, we write: "40:60" = "2:3" (dividing both quantities by 20).
Grammatically, we would say, "40 to 60 equals 2 to 3."
An alternative representation is: "40:60::2:3"
Grammatically, we would say, "40 is to 60 as 2 is to 3."

A ratio that has integers for both quantities and that cannot be reduced any further (using integers) is said to be in simplest form or lowest terms.

Sometimes it is useful to write a ratio in the form 1:n or n:1 to enable comparisons of different ratios.

For example, the ratio 4:5 can be written as 1:1.25 (dividing both sides by 4). Alternatively, 4:5 can be written as 0.8:1 (dividing both sides by 5). Where the context makes the meaning clear, a ratio in this form is sometimes written without the 1 and the colon, though, mathematically, this makes it a factor or multiplier.

Perimeter Area and Volume

Perimeter and Area (2-dimentional shapes)

Perimeter of a shape determines the length around that shape, while the area includes the space inside the shape.

Rectangle:

$P = 2a + 2b$

$A = ab$

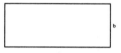

Square

$P = 4a$

$A = a^2$

Parallelogram

$P = 2a + 2b$

$A = ah_a = bh_b$

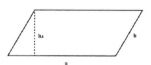

Rhombus

$P = 4a$

$A = ah = \dfrac{d_1 d_2}{2}$

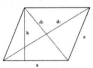

Triangle

$P = a + b + c$

$A = \dfrac{ah_a}{2} = \dfrac{bh_b}{2} = \dfrac{ch_c}{2}$

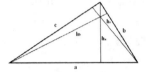

Equilateral Triangle

$P = 3a$

$A = \dfrac{a^2 \sqrt{3}}{4}$

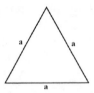

Trapezoid

$P = a + b + c + d$

$A = \dfrac{a + b}{2} h$

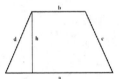

Circle

$P = 2r\pi$

$A = r^2 \pi$

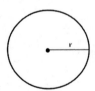

Area and Volume (3-dimentional shapes)

To calculate the area of a 3-dimentional shape, we calculate the areas of all sides and then we add them all.

To find the volume of a 3-dimentional shape, we multiply the area of the base (B) and the height (H) of the 3-dimentional shape.

$$V = BH$$

In case of a pyramid and a cone, the volume would be divided by 3.

$$V = BH/3$$

Here are some of the 3-dimentional shapes with formulas for their area and volume:

Cuboids

$A = 2(ab + bc + ac)$
$V = abc$

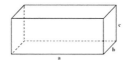

Cube

$A = 6a^2$
$V = a^3$

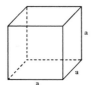

Pyramid

$A = ab + ah_a + bh_b$
$$V = \frac{abH}{3}$$

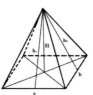

Cylinder

$A = 2r^2\pi + 2r\pi H$
$V = r^2\pi H$

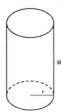

Cone

$A = (r + s)r\pi$
$$V = \frac{r^2\pi H}{3}$$

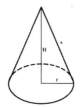

Pythagorean Geometry

If we have a right triangle ABC, where its sides (legs) are a and b and c is a hypotenuse (the side opposite the right angle), then we can establish a relationship between these sides using the following formula:

$$c^2 = a^2 + b^2$$

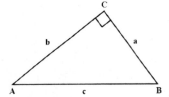

This formula is proven in the Pythagorean Theorem. There are many proofs of this theorem, but we'll look at just one geometrical proof:

If we draw squares on the right triangle's sides, then the area of the square upon the hypotenuse is equal to the sum of the areas of the squares that are upon other two sides of the triangle. Since the areas of these squares are a^2, b^2 and c^2, that is how we got the formula above.

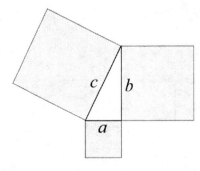

One of the famous right triangles is one with sides 3, 4 and 5. And we can see here that:

$3^2 + 4^2 = 5^2$
$9 + 16 = 25$
$25 = 25$

Example Problem:

The isosceles triangle ABC has a perimeter of 18 centimeters, and the difference between its base and legs is 3 centimeters. Find the height of this triangle.

We write the information we have about triangle ABC and we draw a picture of it for

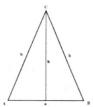

better understanding of the relation between its elements:

P=18 cm
a - b = 3 cm
h=?

We use the formula for the perimeter of the isosceles triangle, since that is what is given to us:

P=a+2b=18 cm

Notice that we have 2 equations with 2 variables, so we can solve it as a system of equations:

a + 2b = 18
a – b = 3 / a + 2b = 18
2a - 2b = 6 / a + 2b + 2a - 2b = 18 + 6
3a = 24
a = 24/3 = 8 cm

Now we go back to find b:
a - b = 3
8 - b = 3
b = 8 - 3
b = 5 cm

Using Pythagorean Theorem, we can find the height using a and b, because the height falls on the side a at the right angle. Notice that height cuts side a exactly in half, and that's why we use in the formula a/2. In this case, b is our hypotenuse, so we have:

$b^2 = (a/2)^2 + h^2$
$h^2 = b^2 - (a/2)^2$
$h^2 = 5^2 - (8/2)^2$
$h^2 = 5^2 - (8/2)^2$
$h^2 = 25 - 4^2$
$h^2 = 26 - 16$
$h^2 = 9$
$h = 3$ cm.

Adding and Subtracting Polynomials

When we are adding or subtracting 2 or more polynomials, we have to first group the same variables (arguments) that have the same degrees and then add or subtract them. For example, if we have ax^3 in one polynomial (where a is some real number), we have to group it with bx^3 from the other polynomial (where b is also some real number). Here is one example with adding polynomials:

$(-x^2 + 2x + 3) + (2x^2 + 4x - 5) =$
$-x^2 + 2x + 3 + 2x^2 + 4x - 5 =$
$x^2 + 6x - 2$

We remove the brackets, and since we have a plus in front of every bracket, the signs in the polynomials don't change.
We group variables with the same degrees. We have $-1 + 2$, which is 1 and that's how we got x^2. For the first degree, where we have $2 + 4$ which is 6, and the constants (real numbers) where we have $3 - 5$ which is -2.

The principle is the same with subtracting, only we have to keep in mind that a minus in front of the polynomial changes all signs in that polynomial. Here is one example:

$(4x^3 - x^2 + 3) - (-3x^2 - 10) =$
$4x^3 - x^2 + 3 + 3x^2 + 10 =$
$4x^3 + 2x^2 + 13$

We remove the brackets, and since we have a minus in front of the second polynomial, all signs in that polynomial change. We have $-3 x^2$ and with minus in front, it becomes a plus and same goes for -10.

Now we group the variables with same degrees: there is no variable with the third degree in the second polynomial, so we just write $4 x^3$. We group other variables the same way as adding polynomials.

Multiplying and Dividing Polynomials

If we have two polynomials that we need to multiply, then multiply each member of the first polynomial with each member of the second. Let's see in one example how this works:

$(x-1)(x-2) = x^2 - 2x - x + 2 = x^2 - 3x + 2$

The first member of the first polynomial is multiplied with the first member of the second polynomial and then with the second member of the second polynomial. Continue the process with the second member of the first polynomial, then simplify.

To multiply more polynomials, multiply the first 2, then multiply that result with next polynomial and so on. Here is one example:

$(1 - x)(2 - x)(3 - x) = (2 - x - 2x + x^2)(3-x)$
$= (2 - 3x + x^2)(3 - x)$
$= 6 - 2x - 9x + 3x^2 + 3x^2 - x^3 = 6 - 11x + 6x^2 - x^3$

Simplifying Polynomials

Let's say we are given some expression with one or more variables, where we have to add, subtract and multiply polynomials. We do the calculations with variables and constants and then we group the variables with the appropriate degrees. As a results, we would get a polynomial. This process is called simplifying polynomials, where we go from a complex expression to a simple polynomial.

Example:

Simplify the following expression and arrange the degrees from bigger to smaller:

$4 + 3x - 2x^2 + 5x + 6x^3 - 2x^2 + 1 = 6x^3 - 4x^2 + 8x + 5$

We can have more complex expressions such as:

$(x + 5)(1 - x) - (2x - 2) = x - x^2 + 5 - 5x - 2x + 2 = -x^2 - 6x + 7$

Here, first we multiply the polynomials and then we subtract the result and the third polynomial.

Factoring Polynomials

If we have a polynomial that we want to write as multiplication of a real number and a polynomial or as a multiplication of 2 or more polynomials, then we are dealing with factoring polynomials.

Let's see an example for a simple factoring:

$12x^2 + 6x - 4 =$
$2 * 6x^2 + 2 * 3x - 2 * 2 =$
$2(6x^2 + 3x - 2)$

We look at every polynomial member as a product of a real number and a variable. Notice that all real numbers in the polynomial are even, so they have the same number (factor). We pull out that 2 in front of the polynomial, and we write what is left.

What if have a more complex case, where we can't find a factor that is a real number? Here is an example:

x² - 2x + 1 =
x² - x - x + 1 =
x(x - 1) - (x - 1) =
(x - 1) (x - 1)

We can write -2x as –x-x . Now we group first 2 members and we see that they have the same factor x, which we can pull in front of them. For the other 2 members, we pull the minus in front of them, so we can get the same binomial that we got with the first 2 members. Now we have that this binomial is the factor for x(x-1) and (x-1).
If we pull x-1 in front (underlined), from the first member we are left with x, and from the second we have -1.
And that is how we transform a polynomial into a product of 2 polynomials (in this case binomials).

Quadratic equations

A. Factoring

Quadratic equations are usually called second degree equations, which mean that the second degree is the highest degree of the variable that can be found in the quadratic equation. The form of these equations is:

$$ax^2 + bx + c = 0$$

where a, b and c are some real numbers.

One way for solving quadratic equations is the factoring method, where we transform the quadratic equation into a product of 2 or more polynomials. Let's see how that works in one simple example:

$$x^2 + 2x = 0$$

$$x(x + 2) = 0$$

$$(x = 0) \vee (x + 2 = 0)$$

$$(x = 0) \vee (x = -2)$$

Notice that here we don't have parameter c, but this is still a quadratic equation, because we have the second degree of variable x. Our factor here is x, which we put in front and we are left with x+2. The equation is equal to 0, so either x or x+2 are 0, or both are 0.
So, our 2 solutions are 0 and -2.

B. Quadratic formula
If we are unsure how to rewrite quadratic equations so we can solve it using factoring method, we can use the formula for quadratic equation:

$$x_{1,2} = \frac{-b \pm \sqrt{b^2 - 4ac}}{2a}$$

We write $x_{1,2}$ because it represents 2 solutions of the equation. Here is one example:

$3x^2 - 10x + 3 = 0$

$x_{1,2} = \frac{-b \pm \sqrt{b^2 - 4ac}}{2a}$

$x_{1,2} = \frac{-(-10) \pm \sqrt{(-10)^2 - 4 \cdot 3 \cdot 3}}{2 \cdot 3}$

$x_{1,2} = \frac{10 \pm \sqrt{100 - 36}}{6}$

$x_{1,2} = \frac{10 \pm \sqrt{64}}{6}$

$x_{1,2} = \frac{10 \pm 8}{6}$

$x_1 = \frac{10 + 8}{6} = \frac{18}{6} = 3$

$x_2 = \frac{10 - 8}{6} = \frac{2}{6} = \frac{1}{3}$

We see that a is 3, b is -10 and c is 3.
We use these numbers in the equation and do some calculations.

Notice that we have + and -, so x_1 is for + and x_2 is for -, and that's how we get 2 solutions.

Momentum

Momentum can be described as the sum product of the mass of an object and its velocity. This means that momentum measures the force produced by an object's mass and velocity.
The formula for calculating momentum is =
Momentum = mass X velocity
Or
P = MV
Where P = momentum, V = velocity and M = mass

Based on the above definition, it is clear that the momentum of a car and a bicycle both travelling at 20 m/s will not be the same, because although the velocity of the two objects are the same, their mass is different. The car would have greater momentum, due to its larger mass.

It is important to note that:

The SI unit for velocity = m/s
SI unit for Mass = kg
So therefore momentum = kg x m/s and SI unit for momentum is kg x m/s

Momentum must always have a direction and so the final answer must reflect the direction of the momentum or velocity.

Sample questions

1
Find the momentum of a round stone weighing 12.05 kg rolling down a hill at 8m/s.

Formula - P= kg x m/s
= 12.05kg x 8m/s
= 96.4 kg x m/s down hill

Take note that the final answer has the proper SI unit of momentum (kg x m/s) after it and it also mentions the direction of the movement.

2
A cannon ball weighing 35kg is shot from a cannon towards the east at 220mls, calculate the momentum of the cannon ball.

Formula - P= kg x m/s
= 35kg x 220m/s
= 7700 kg x m/s east

Science

This section contains a science self-assessment and tutorials. The Tutorials are designed to familiarize general principals and the self-assessment contains general questions similar to the science questions likely to be on the PAX RN exam, but are not intended to be identical to the exam questions. Many Universities recommend that students take an introductory Science course before taking the PAX RN Exam. The tutorials are *not* designed to be a complete science course, and it is assumed that students have some familiarity with Science. If you do not understand parts of the tutorial, or find the tutorial difficult, it is recommended that you seek out additional instruction.

Tour of the PAX RN Science Content

The PAX RN science section currently has 100 science questions which cover Biology, Chemistry, Anatomy and Physiology and Physics. The Physics component is currently being tested and is not given at all institutions. Be sure to check with your school for the exact content of the exam you will be taking. Below is a detailed list of the science topics likely to appear on the PAX RN. Anatomy and Physiology questions are reviewed in detail in the next chapter. Make sure that you understand these at the very minimum.

Biology

- Cellular processes

- Scientific reasoning and scientific method

- Classification and Taxonomy

- Photosynthesis

- Genetics

Chemistry

- Atoms and molecules

- Protons and electrons

- States of matter

- Redox reactions

- Chemical reactions

- Acid and base

- Molarity

- Periodic table

Physics

- Potential, mechanical and kinetic energy

- Electricity - currents voltage and resistance

- Ohm's law

- Newton's laws

- Linear and rotational motion

The questions below are not exactly the same as you will find on the PAX RN - that would be too easy! And nobody knows what the questions will be and they change all the time. Mostly the changes consist of substituting new questions for old, but the changes also can be new question formats or styles, changes to the number of questions in each section, changes to the time limits for each section and combing sections. Below are general Science questions that cover the same areas as the PAX RN. So while the format and exact wording of the questions may differ slightly, and changes from year to year, if you can answer the questions below, you will have no problem with the Science section of the PAX RN.

Science Self Assessment

The purpose of the self-assessment is:

- Identify your strengths and weaknesses.

- Develop your personalized study plan (above)

- Get accustomed to the PAX RN format

- Extra practice – the self-assessment is a 3rd test!

- Provide a baseline score for preparing your study schedule.

Since this is a self-assessment, and depending on how confident you are with basic science, timing yourself is optional. The biology, chemistry and optional physics sections have 75 questions to be answered in 75 minutes. The self-assessment has 40 questions, so allow 50 minutes to complete.

Once complete, use the table below to assess you understanding of the content, and prepare your study schedule described in chapter 1.

80% - 100%	Excellent – you have mastered the content
60% – 79%	Good. You have a working knowledge. Even though you can just pass this section, you may want to review the tutorials and do some extra practice to see if you can improve your mark.
40% - 59%	Below Average. You do not understand the content. Review the tutorials, and retake this quiz again in a few days, before proceeding to the Practice Test Questions.
Less than 40%	Poor. You have a very limited understanding of the content. Please review the tutorials, and retake this quiz again in a few days, before proceeding to the Practice Test Questions.

Science Self Assessment Answer Sheet

1. Ⓐ Ⓑ Ⓒ Ⓓ   11. Ⓐ Ⓑ Ⓒ Ⓓ   21. Ⓐ Ⓑ Ⓒ Ⓓ

2. Ⓐ Ⓑ Ⓒ Ⓓ   12. Ⓐ Ⓑ Ⓒ Ⓓ   22. Ⓐ Ⓑ Ⓒ Ⓓ

3. Ⓐ Ⓑ Ⓒ Ⓓ   13. Ⓐ Ⓑ Ⓒ Ⓓ   23. Ⓐ Ⓑ Ⓒ Ⓓ

4. Ⓐ Ⓑ Ⓒ Ⓓ   14. Ⓐ Ⓑ Ⓒ Ⓓ   24. Ⓐ Ⓑ Ⓒ Ⓓ

5. Ⓐ Ⓑ Ⓒ Ⓓ   15. Ⓐ Ⓑ Ⓒ Ⓓ   25. Ⓐ Ⓑ Ⓒ Ⓓ

6. Ⓐ Ⓑ Ⓒ Ⓓ   16. Ⓐ Ⓑ Ⓒ Ⓓ

7. Ⓐ Ⓑ Ⓒ Ⓓ   17. Ⓐ Ⓑ Ⓒ Ⓓ

8. Ⓐ Ⓑ Ⓒ Ⓓ   18. Ⓐ Ⓑ Ⓒ Ⓓ

9. Ⓐ Ⓑ Ⓒ Ⓓ   19. Ⓐ Ⓑ Ⓒ Ⓓ

10. Ⓐ Ⓑ Ⓒ Ⓓ   20. Ⓐ Ⓑ Ⓒ Ⓓ

Physics

1. Which of the following is not true of atomic theory?

a. Originated in the early 19th century with the work of John Dalton.

b. Is the field of physics that describes the characteristics and properties of atoms that make up matter.

c. Explains temperature as the momentum of atoms.

d. Explains macroscopic phenomenon through the behavior of microscopic atoms.

2. Which of these statements about atoms is/are incorrect?

a. Are the largest unit of matter that can take part in a chemical reaction.

b. Can be chemically broken down into much simpler forms.

c. Are composed of protons and neutrons in a central nucleus surrounded by electrons.

d. Do not differ in terms of atomic number or atomic mass.

3. Protons, neutrons, and electrons differ in that:

a. Protons and neutrons form the nucleus of an atom, while electrons are found in fixed energy levels around the nucleus of the atom.

b. Protons and neutrons are charged particles and electrons are neutral.

c. Protons and neutrons form fixed energy levels around the nucleus of the atom and electrons are located near the surface of the atom.

d. Protons, neutrons and electrons are charged particles.

4. Newton's laws of motion consist of three physical laws that form the basis for classical mechanics. Which of the following is/are not included in these laws?

a. Unless acted upon by a force, a body at rest stays at rest.

b. Unless acted upon by a force, a body in motion will change direction and gradually slow until it eventually stops.

c. To every action, there is an equal and opposite reaction.

d. A body acted upon by a force will accelerate in the same direction as the force at a magnitude that is directly proportional to the force.

5. A car starts from a full top and in 20 seconds is travelling 10/m per second. What is the acceleration?

    a. $0.5 \ m/sec^2$

    b. $0.24 \ m/sec^2$

    c. $1 \ m/sec^2$

    d. $1.5 \ m/sec^2$

6. The space station travels 1000 meters in 5 seconds. How fast is it travelling?

    a. 100 meters/second

    b. 200 meters/second

    c. 50 meters/second

    d. 500 meters/second

7. How much force is needed to accelerate a car weighing 2,000 kg, at a rate of $3 \ m/s^2$?

    a. 6000 N

    b. 3000 N

    c. 2000 N

    d. 1000 N

8. Protons, neutrons, and electrons differ in that:

    a. Protons and neutrons form the nucleus of an atom, while electrons are found in fixed energy levels around the nucleus of the atom.

    b. Protons and neutrons are charged particles and electrons are neutral.

    c. Protons and neutrons form fixed energy levels around the nucleus of the atom and electrons are located near the surface of the atom.

    d. Protons, neutrons and electrons are charged particles.

Biology

9. Classification is a grouping of organisms based on similar

    a. Traits and evolutionary histories

    b. Traits and biological histories

    c. Behaviors and evolutionary histories

    d. Traits and evolutionary advancement

10. A method for categorizing organisms by their biological type is known as:

  a. Anatomical classification.

  b. Biological classification.

  c. Physical classification.

  d. Cellular classification.

11. When compared to homologous traits, "analogous" traits refer to ones that:

  a. Are similar but the similarity does not derive from a common ancestor.

  b. Are similar because they had the same parents.

  c. Are not similar and do not come from a common ancestor.

  d. Are completely equal.

12. Which, if any, of the following statements about mitosis are correct?

  a. Mitosis is the process of cell division by which identical daughter cells are produced.

  b. Following mitosis, new cells contain less DNA than did the original cells.

  c. During mitosis, the chromosome number is doubled.

  d. A and C are correct.

13. What is a nucleic acid that carries the genetic information in the cell and is capable of self-replication?

  a. RNA

  b. Triglyceride

  c. DNA

  d. DAR

14. The segment of a DNA molecule determining the amino acid sequence of protein is known as

  a. Operator gene

  b. Structural gene

  c. Regulator gene

  d. Modifier gene

15. Cells that line the inner or outer surfaces of organs or body cavities are often linked together by intimate physical connections. What are these connections?

    a. Separate desmosomes

    b. Ronofilaments

    c. Tight junctions

    d. Fascia adherenes

16. Genes control heredity in man and other organisms. These genes are

    a. A segment of RNA or DNA

    b. A bead like structure on the chromosomes

    c. A protein molecule

    d. A segment of RNA

17. Who was a 19th century scientist who outlined the original theory of inheritance?

    a. Albert Einstein

    b. Christian Doppler

    c. Gregor Mendel

    d. Charles Darwin

18. Describe the science of genetics.

    a. Is a branch of biology concerned with the study of heredity and variation.

    b. Attempts to explain how characteristics of living organisms are passed on from one generation to the next.

    c. Is a measure of the variety of the of the Earth's animal, plant, and microbial species.

    d. A and B

19. Describe enzymes

    a. Most enzymes are proteins that are selective catalysts

    b. Enzymes are catalysts that accelerate metabolic reactions

    c. Enzymes are chemical agents that assist metabolic reactions

    d. Enzymes are biological agents that decrease the rate of reaction

Chemistry

20. In the periodic table of the elements, elements are arranged in order of their atomic _____, which is the number of _____ found in their nucleus.

  a. Mass, protons

  b. Number, neutrons

  c. Mass, neutrons

  d. Number, protons

21. What are the differences, if any, between mixtures and compounds?

  a. A mixture is homogeneous, and the properties of its components are retained, while a compound is heterogeneous and its properties are distinct from those of the elements combined in its formation.

  b. A mixture is heterogeneous, and the properties of its components are retained, while a compound is homogeneous and its properties are distinct from those of the elements combined in its formation.

  c. A mixture is heterogeneous, and the properties of its components are changed, while a compound is homogeneous and its properties are similar to those of the elements combined in its formation.

  d. A compound is heterogeneous, and the properties of its components are retained, while a mixture is homogeneous and its properties are distinct from those of the elements combined in its formation.

22. What are the differences, if any, between chemical changes and physical changes?

  a. During a physical change, some aspect of the physical properties of matter are altered, but the identity of the substance remains constant. Chemical changes involve the alteration of both a substance's composition and structure.

  b. During a chemical change, some aspect of the physical properties of matter are altered, but the identity of the substance remains constant. Physical changes involve the alteration of both a substance's composition and structure.

  c. During a physical change, no aspects of the physical properties of matter are altered, but the identity of the substance remains constant. Chemical changes involve the alteration of both a substance's composition and structure.

  d. There is no substantive difference between chemical and physical changes.

23. A _____ is a process that transforms one set of chemical substances to another; the substances used are known as _____ and those formed are _____.

    a. A chemical change is a process that transforms one set of chemical substances to another; the substances used are known as products and those formed are reactants.

    b. A biological change is a process that transforms one set of chemical substances to another; the substances used are known as reactants and those formed are products.

    c. A chemical change is a process that transforms one set of chemical substances to another; the substances used are known as reactants and those formed are products.

    A chemical variation is a process that transforms one set of chemical substances to another; the substances used are known as reactants and those formed are products.

24. _____ is the most abundant element in the Earth's crust and appears on the Atomic Table as the letter ____.

    a. Nitrogen, N

    b. Oxygen, O

    c. Silicon, Si

    d. Sodium, Na

25. In the periodic table the elements are arranged in

    a. Order of increasing atomic number

    b. Alphabetical order

    c. Order of increasing metallic properties

    d. Order of increasing neutron content

26. The molarity of 5 liters of a salt solution is 0.5 M of salt solution. Calculate the moles of salt in the solution.

    a. 1

    b. 2

    c. 2.5

    d. 3

Scientific Reasoning

27. In science, _____ is defined as a difference between the desired and actual performance or behavior of a system or object.

    a. Accuracy

    b. Uncertainty

    c. Error

    d. Mistake

28. When employing the scientific method of research, the researcher follows these steps:

    a. Define the question, make observations, offer a possible explanation, perform an experiment, analyze data, draw conclusions.

    b. Make observations, offer a possible explanation, define the question, perform an experiment, analyze, draw conclusions.

    c. Perform an experiment, make observations, define the question, offer a possible explanation, analyze the data, draw conclusions.

    d. Make observations, define the question, offer a possible explanation, perform an experiment, analyze data, draw conclusions.

29. What is the principle that generally advises choosing the competing hypothesis that makes the fewest new assumptions, when the hypotheses are equal in other respects?

    a. Hickam's Dictum

    b. Boyle's Law

    c. Dalton's Law

    d. Occam's Razor

30. A _____ _____ is a statistic used as a measure of the dispersion or variation in a distribution.

    a. Normal distribution

    b. Range

    c. Outlier

    d. Standard deviation

Answer Key

1. C
Answer c is incorrect because atomic theory explains temperature as the motion of atoms (faster = hotter), not the momentum. The momentum of atoms explains the outward pressure that they exert.

2. D
The atoms of different elements differ in atomic number, relative atomic mass, and chemical behavior

3. A
Protons and neutrons form the nucleus of an atom, while electrons are found in fixed energy levels around the nucleus of the atom.

4. B
Unless acted upon by a force, a body in motion will change direction and gradually slow until it eventually stops.

This answer is related to Newton's 1st law of motion that states that, unless acted upon by a force, a body at rest stays at rest, and a moving body continues moving at the same speed in a straight line.

5. A
The formula for acceleration = $A = (V_f - V_0)/t$
so $A = (10 \text{ m/sec} - 0 \text{ m/sec})/20 \text{ sec} = 0.5 \text{ m/sec}^2$

6. B
Speed = (total distance traveled)/(total time taken)
1000/5 = 200 meters per second

7. A
Force = Mass times Acceleration Measured in Newtons.
$F = 2000 \text{ kg} \times 3 \text{ m/sec}^2 = 6000 \text{ N}$

8. A
Protons and neutrons form the nucleus of an atom, while electrons are found in fixed energy levels around the nucleus of the atom.

Biology

9. A
Classification is a grouping of organisms based on similar traits and evolutionary histories.

Note: Taxonomy and systematics are the two sciences that attempt to classify living things. In taxonomy, organisms are assigned to groups based on their characteristics. In modern systematics, the placement of organisms into groups is based on evolutionary relationships.

10. B

Biological classification. Classification is more a matter of convenience; in reality, there are many times when the various classifications tend to blur into one another.

11. A

Analogous traits are similar but the similarity does not derive from a common ancestor.

12. A and C are correct.

a. Mitosis is the process of cell division by which identical daughter cells are produced.

c. During mitosis, the chromosome number is doubled.

13. C

DNA is a nucleic acid that carries the genetic information in the cell and is capable of self-replication.

14. B

A structural gene is the segment of a DNA molecule determining the amino acid sequence of protein. DNA is a nucleic acid that contains the genetic instructions used in the development and functioning of all known living organisms (with the exception of RNA viruses). The DNA segments that carry this genetic information are called genes but other DNA sequences have structural purposes or are involved in regulating the use of this genetic information. Along with RNA and proteins DNA is one of the three major macromolecules that are essential for all known forms of life.

15. C

Tight junctions or zonula occludens are the closely associated areas of two cells whose membranes join together forming a virtually impermeable barrier to fluid. It is a type of junctional complex present only in vertebrates. The corresponding junctions that occur in invertebrates are septate junctions. [4]

16. A

Genes are made from a long molecule called DNA which is copied and inherited across generations. DNA is made of simple units that line up in a particular order within this large molecule. The order of these units carries genetic information similar to how the order of letters on a page carries information. The language used by DNA is called the genetic code which lets organisms read the information in the genes. This information is the instructions for constructing and operating a living organism.

17. C

Gregor Mendel was a 19th century scientist who outlined the original theory of inheritance.

18. D

A and B describe genetics.

a. Is a branch of biology concerned with the study of heredity and variation.

b. Attempts to explain how characteristics of living organisms are passed on from one generation to the next.

19. A

Most enzymes are proteins that are selective catalysts

Chemistry

20. D

In the Periodic Table, elements are arranged in order of their atomic number, which is the number of protons found in their nucleus.

21. B

A mixture is heterogeneous, and the properties of its components are retained, while a compound is homogeneous and its properties are distinct from those of the elements combined in its formation.

22. A

During a physical change, some aspect of the physical properties of matter are altered, but the identity of the substance remains constant. Chemical changes involve the alteration of both a substance's composition and structure.

23. C

A chemical change is a process that transforms one set of chemical substances to another; the substances used are known as reactants and those formed are products.

24. B

Oxygen is the most abundant element in the Earth's crust and appears on the Atomic Table as the letter O.

25. A

The periodic table of the chemical elements (also known as the periodic table or periodic table of the elements) is a tabular display of the 118 known chemical elements organized by selected properties of their atomic structures. Elements are presented by increasing atomic number, the number of protons in an atom's atomic nucleus.

26. C

Moles of solute = ? or X
Solutions liters = 5 liters
Molarity of solution = 0.5 M

Therefore: X moles/5 liters of solution = 0.5 or X/5 = 0.5
So X = 5/0.5
X = 2.5

Scientific Method and Reasoning

27. C
In science, Error is defined as a difference between the desired and actual performance or behavior of a system or object.

28. A
When employing the scientific method of research, the researcher follows these steps: define the question, make observations, offer a possible explanation, perform an experiment, analyze data, draw conclusions.

29. D
Occam's Razor is a principle that generally advises choosing the competing hypothesis that makes the fewest new assumptions, when the hypotheses are equal in other respects.

30. D
A Standard deviation is a statistic used as a measure of the dispersion or variation in a distribution.

Science Tutorials

Scientific Method

The scientific method is a set of steps that allow people who ask "how" and "why" questions about the world to go about finding valid answers that accurately reflect reality.

Were it not for the scientific method, people would have no valid method for drawing quantifiable and accurate information about the world.

There are four primary steps to the scientific method:

1. Analyzing an aspect of reality and asking "how" or "why" it works or exists
2. Forming a hypothesis that explains "how" or "why"
3. Making a prediction about the sort of things that would happen if the hypothesis were true
4. Performing an experiment to test your prediction.

These steps vary somewhat depending on the field of science you happen to be studying. (In astronomy, for instance, experiments are generally eschewed in favor of observational evidence confirming that predictions are true.) But for the most part this is the model scientists follow.

Observation and Analysis

The first step in the scientific method requires you to determine what it is about reality that you want to explore.

You might notice that your friends who eat regular servings of fruits and vegetables are healthier and more athletic than your friends who live off red meat and meals covered in cheese and gravy. This is an observation and, noting it, you are likely to ask yourself "why" it seems to be true. At this stage of the scientific method, scientists will often do research to see if anyone else has explored similar observations and analyze what other people's findings have been. This is an important step not only because it can show you what others have found to be true about their observation, but because it can show what others have found to be false, which can be equally as valuable.

Hypothesis

After making your observation and doing some research, you can form your hypothesis. A hypothesis is an idea you formulate based on the evidence you have already gathered about "how" your observation relates to reality.

Using the example of your friends' diets, you may have found research discussing vitamin levels in fruits and vegetables and how certain vitamins will affect a person's health and athleticism. This research may lead you to hypothesize that the foods your healthy friends are eating contain specific types of vitamins, and it is the vitamins making them healthy. Just as importantly, however, is applying research that shows hypotheses that were later proven wrong. Scientists need to know this information, too, as it can help keep them from making errors in their thinking. For instance, you could come across a research paper in which someone hypothesized that the sugars in fruits and vegetables gave people more energy, which then helped them be more athletic. If the paper were to go on to explain that no such link was found, and that the protein and carbohydrates in meat and gravy contained far more energy than the sugar, you would know that this hypothesis was wrong and that there was no need for you to waste time exploring it.

Prediction

The third step in the scientific method is making a prediction based on your hypothesis.

Forming predictions is vital to the scientific method because if your prediction turns out to be correct, it will demonstrate that your hypothesis can accurately explain some aspect of the world. This is important because one aspect of the scientific method is its ability to prove objectively that your way of understanding the world is valid. We can take the simple example of a car that will not start. If you notice the fuel gauge is pointing towards empty, you can announce your prediction to the other passengers that a careful test of the gas tank will show the car has no fuel. While this seems obvious, it is still important to note since a prediction like this is the only way to really *prove* to your friends that you understand how a fuel gauge works and what it means.
In the same way a prediction made by a hypothesis is the only way to really show that it represents reality. For instance, based on your vitamin hypothesis you may predict people can be healthy and athletic while eating whatever they want as long as they take vitamin supplements. If this prediction ends up being true, it will show that it is in fact the vitamins, and only the vitamins, in fruits and vegetables that make people healthy and athletic. It will prove that your hypothesis shows how vitamins work.

Experiment

The final step is to perform an experiment that tests your prediction.

You may decide to separate your healthy friends into three groups, give one group vitamin supplements and prohibit them from eating vegetables, give another fake supplements and prohibit them from eating vegetables and have the third act normally as the control group. It is always important to have a control group so you have someone acting "normally" to compare your results against. If this experiment shows the real supplement group and the control group maintaining the same level of health and athleticism while the fake supplement group grows weak and sickly, you will know your hypothesis is true. If, on the other hand, you get unexpected results, you will need to go back to step one, analyze your results, make new observations and try again with a different hypothesis.

Any hypothesis that cannot be confirmed with experiment (or in the case of fields such as astronomy, with observation) cannot be considered true and must be altered or abandoned. It is in this stage where scientists—being humans, with human beliefs and prejudices—are most likely to abandon the scientific method. If an experiment or observation gives a scientist results that he or she does not like, the scientist may be inclined to ignore the results rather than reexamine the hypothesis. This was the case for nearly a thousand years in astronomy with astronomers attempting to form accurate models of the solar system based on circular orbits of the planets and on Earth being in the center. For philosophical reasons it was believed that circles were "perfect" and that the Earth was "important," so no model that had the correct elliptical orbits or the sun properly in the center was accepted until the 16th century, even though those models more accurately described all astronomers' observations.

Biology

Biology is a natural science concerned with the study of life and living organisms, including their structure, function, growth, origin, evolution, distribution, and taxonomy.

Biology is a vast subject containing many subdivisions, topics, and disciplines. Among the most important topics are five unifying principles that can be said to be the fundamental axioms of modern biology:

- Cells are the basic unit of life

- New species and inherited traits are the product of evolution

- Genes are the basic unit of heredity

- An organism regulates its internal environment to maintain a stable and constant condition

- Living organisms consume and transform energy.

Sub-disciplines of biology are recognized on the basis of the scale at which organisms are studied and the methods used to study them: biochemistry examines the rudimentary chemistry of life; molecular biology studies the complex interactions of systems of biological molecules; cellular biology examines the basic building block of all life, the cell; physiology examines the physical and chemical functions of the tissues, organs, and organ systems of an organism; and ecology examines how various organisms interact and associate with their environment. [5]

Cell Biology

Cell biology (formerly cytology, from the Greek kytos, "contain") is a scientific discipline that studies cells – their physiological properties, their structure, the organelles they contain, interactions with their environment, their life cycle, division and death.

This is done both on a microscopic and molecular level. Cell biology research encompasses both the great diversity of single-celled organisms like bacteria and protozoa, as well as the many specialized cells in multicellular organisms such as humans.

Knowing the components of cells and how cells work is fundamental to all biological sciences.

Appreciating the similarities and differences between cell types is particularly important to the fields of cell and molecular biology as well as to biomedical fields such as cancer research and developmental biology. These fundamental similarities and differences provide a unifying theme, sometimes allowing the principles learned from studying one cell type to be extrapolated and generalized to other cell types. Therefore, research in cell biology is closely related to genetics, biochemistry, molecular biology, immunology, and developmental biology.

Each type of protein is usually sent to a particular part of the cell.

An important part of cell biology is the investigation of molecular mechanisms by which proteins are moved to different places inside cells or secreted from cells.

Processes – Movement of Proteins

Most proteins are synthesized by ribosomes in the rough endoplasmic reticulum.

Ribosomes contain the nucleic acid RNA, which assembles and joins amino acids to make proteins. They can be found alone or in groups within the cytoplasm as well as on the RER.

This process is known as protein biosynthesis.

Biosynthesis (also called biogenesis) is an enzyme-catalyzed process in cells of living organisms by which substrates are converted to more complex products (also simply known as protein translation). Some proteins, such as those to be incorporated in membranes (known as membrane proteins), are transported into the "rough" endoplasmic reticulum (ER) during synthesis. This process can be followed by transportation and processing in the Golgi apparatus.

The Golgi apparatus is a large organelle that processes proteins and prepares them for use both inside and outside the cell.

The Golgi apparatus is somewhat like a post office. It receives items (proteins from the ER), packages and labels them, and then sends them on to their destinations (to different parts of the cell or to the cell membrane for transport out of the cell). From the Golgi, membrane proteins can move to the plasma membrane, to other sub-cellular compartments, or they can be secreted from the cell.

The ER and Golgi can be thought of as the "membrane protein synthesis compartment" and the "membrane protein processing compartment", respectively.

There is a semi-constant flux of proteins through these compartments. ER and Golgi-resident proteins associate with other proteins but remain in their respective compartments. Other proteins "flow" through the ER and Golgi to the plasma membrane. Motor proteins transport membrane protein-containing vesicles along cytoskeletal tracks to distant parts of cells such as axon terminals.

Some proteins that are made in the cytoplasm contain structural features that target them for transport into mitochondria or the nucleus.

Some mitochondrial proteins are made inside mitochondria and are coded for by mitochondrial DNA. In plants, chloroplasts also make some cell proteins.

Extracellular and cell surface proteins destined to be degraded can move back into intracellular compartments upon being incorporated into endocytosed vesicles some of which fuse with lysosomes where the proteins are broken down to their individual amino acids. The degradation of some membrane proteins begins while still at the cell surface when they are separated by secretases. Proteins that function in the cytoplasm are often degraded by proteasomes.

Other cellular processes

Active and Passive transport - Movement of molecules into and out of cells.
Autophagy - The process whereby cells "eat" their own internal components or microbial invaders.
Adhesion - Holding together cells and tissues.
Reproduction - Made possible by the combination of sperm made in the testiculi (contained in some male cells' nuclei) and the egg made in the ovary (contained in the nucleus of a female cell). When the sperm breaks through the hard outer shell of the

egg a new cell embryo is formed, which, in humans, grows to full size in 9 months.
Cell movement - Chemotaxis, Contraction, cilia and flagella.
Cell signalling - Regulation of cell behavior by signals from outside.
DNA repair and Cell death
Metabolism - Glycolysis, respiration, Photosynthesis
Transcription and mRNA splicing - gene expression.

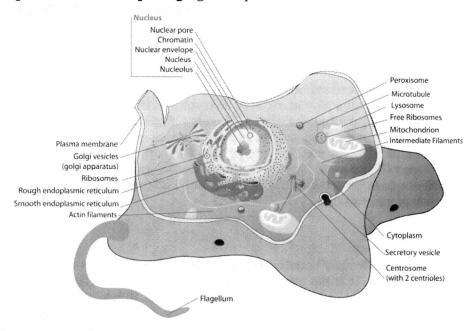

6

Internal cellular structures

Chloroplast - key organelle for photosynthesis (only found in plant cells)
Cilia - motile microtubule-containing structures of eukaryotes
Cytoplasm - contents of the main fluid-filled space inside cells
Cytoskeleton - protein filaments inside cells
Endoplasmic reticulum - major site of membrane protein synthesis
Flagella - motile structures of bacteria, archaea and eukaryotes
Golgi apparatus - site of protein glycosylation in the endomembrane system
Lipid bilayer - fundamental organizational structure of cell membranes
Lysosome - break down cellular waste products and debris into simple compounds (only found in animal cells)
Membrane lipid and protein barrier
Mitochondrion - major energy-producing organelle by releasing it in the form of ATP
Nucleus - holds most of the DNA of eukaryotic cells and controls all cellular activities
Organelle - term used for major subcellular structures
Ribosome - RNA and protein complex required for protein synthesis in cells
Vesicle - small membrane-bounded spheres inside cells

Chromosomes, genes, proteins, RNA and DNA

The concepts of genes, chromosomes, proteins, RNA and DNA are all interrelated genetic terms. Chromosomes are made up of genes, the DNA contains the chromosomes and the RNA interprets and implements the information in the RNA. Here is a break down of each of them.

Proteins

Proteins are biological molecules that are made up of a chain or chains of amino acids. Proteins play many very vital roles in living organisms. Protein is essential for the performance of many bodily functions such as replicating DNA, transporting nutrients and molecules within the body, responding to stimuli, and acting as a catalyst for metabolic reactions within the living organism, among other things. There are different types of proteins and they play various roles. The difference in proteins would be determined by their unique arrangement or sequence of amino acids.

Genes

A gene is the molecular hereditary unity of an organism and a small part of the chromosome. It is the term used to describe a portion of RNA or DNA code that performs a particular function in the organism. Genes are essential to life because they specify the functions of all proteins and RNA chains. Genes contain the information to maintain and build the cells in the organism and also contain genetic information that would be passed on to the offspring.

Genes hold the information for biological traits and functions some of which can clearly be seen and some of which are hidden. For example, the information contained in specific genes determines factors such as eye color, hair color, number of limbs, height and so on. Some traits such as blood type and the thousands of metabolic reactions and biochemical process that take place in the body to sustain life are defined unseen by the genes.

A gene is set of basic instruction embedded on a sequence of nucleic acids. The gene is a locatable region of the DNA genome sequence that correspond to a unit of inheritance and associated with a particular body function or set of functions.

Chromosomes

The chromosome is a piece of the DNA containing several genes. The chromosome is an organized part of the DNA. It is a single piece of coiled DNA. The chromosome contains several genes, DNA-bound proteins, nucleotide sequences and regulatory elements. The DNA-bound proteins help to hold the DNA together and regulate its functions.

Since the chromosomes contain the genes, they contain almost all the genetic information of the organism. Chromosomes differ from one organism to another.

The DNA molecule could be linear or circular. The chromosome can contain from 100,000 to over 3 million nucleotides in one long chain depending on the organism. Cells with defined nuclei (eukaryotic cells) usually have large linear shaped chromosomes. Cells without clearly defined nuclei (prokaryotic cells) usually have smaller sized circular chromosomes.

Chromosomes are essential in the process of cell division. In mitosis cell division, the chromosomes have to be replicated and then divided among the two resulting daughter cells. This ensures that the resulting two daughter cells are genetically identical to the original mother cell.

DNA

DNA or Deoxyribonucleic acid is an essential component of life. It has been described as the blueprint of a living organism. It contains vital genetic information and instructions that are required for the proper functioning and development of all types and forms of living organisms and even viruses. DNA, proteins and RNA are the three most important macro-molecules that are essential for any form of life.

The genetic information contained in the DNA is encoded as a sequence of nucleotides known as G, A, and C. With G being guanine, A adenine, T thymine and C cytosine. These nucleotides are arranged as DNA molecules in a double-stranded helix. The strands run in opposite directions and are thus anti-parallel. The DNA contains long structures known as chromosomes.

RNA

RNA or Ribonucleic acids are large biological molecules that perform the important roles of decoding, coding, regulating and expressing the genes and the information contained within them. RNA, DNA and proteins are three essential components for all form of life. The RNA is also composed of nucleotides, but unlike the DNA that is double stranded, the RNA is single stranded.

In organisms, some RNA components serve as messengers to convey genetic information to direct the synthesis or use of specific proteins for specific purposes. It can thus be said that RNA is essential for the proper carrying out of the information contained in the DNA genes. RNA plays important roles within the cell such as helping to catalyze biological reactions sense and communicate cellular signals and control gene expressions. RNA is also essential for protein synthesis.

Classification

Classification

Taxonomic classification is the primary method of organizing the Earth's biology. Taxonomy means,

1. The classification of organisms in an ordered system that indicates natural relationships.
2. The science, laws, or principles of classification

The earliest form of classification that bears any resemblance to the current system can be traced back to ancient Greece with Aristotle's organization of animals based on reproduction.

The classification into kingdoms (animal, mineral and vegetable) was developed by Carolus Linnaeus.

The true father of modern taxonomical classification, however, is Carolus Linnaeus, who in the early 18th century developed a system of kingdoms that separated life into the categories animal, mineral and vegetable. Although Linnaeus's work lacked what would today be considered essential technologies (such as microscopes capable of imaging bacteria) and theories (such as evolution), much of his system has survived in modern classification.

Charles Darwin's theory of evolution was an important factor in taxonomic classification.

With Charles Darwin's publication of On the Origin of Species in 1859 the evolutionary process became a major factor in taxonomic classification. For the first time biology could be classified by grouping the direct descendents of common ancestors rather than just grouping creatures with similar characteristics.

The main classifications are, domain, kingdom, phylum, class, order, family, genus and species.

Today, the majority of scientists accept a hierarchical structuring of biology that goes from general, or large, to specific: domain, kingdom, phylum, class, order, family, genus and species. (There are sometimes smaller subcategories such as superfamily, subfamily, tribe and subspecies listed, but these are the primary eight categories.) Domain is the newest of these and is split into three primary groups: Bacteria, Archaea and Eukarya.
Each of these domains is split again with Bacteria splitting into the Kingdom Bacteria, Archaea splitting into the Kingdom Archaea and Eukarya splitting into the four kingdoms of Protista, Plantae, Fungi and finally our kingdom, Animalia. The Domain Eukarya splits so many times because eukaryotic cells are highly complex, containing such important features as cell walls and nuclei.

As a result of this complexity, eukaryotic cells have gone through a much more diverse evolutionary process than prokaryotic cells such as bacteria and archaea, and thus Eukarya make up all complex life on Earth

Rank	Fruit fly	Human	Pea	*E. coli*
Domain	Eukarya	Eukarya	Eukarya	Bacteria
Kingdom	Animalia	Animalia	Plantae	Bacteria
Phylum or **Division**	Arthropoda	Chordata	Magnoliophyta	
Subphylum or subdivision	Hexapoda	Vertebrata		
Class	Insecta	Mammalia	Magnoliopsida	
Subclass	Pterygota	Theria	Rosidae	
Order	Diptera	Primates	Fabales	
Suborder	Brachycera		Fabineae	
Family	Drosophilidae	Hominidae	Fabaceae	
Subfamily	Drosophilinae	Homininae	Faboideae	
Genus	*Drosophila*	*Homo*	*Pisum*	*Escherichia*
Species	*D. melanogaster*	*H. sapiens*	*P. sativum*	*E. coli*

7

Each Kingdom has a huge number of organisms. Bacteria and Archaea (single celled organisms).

Within each of the kingdoms the number of creatures is far too many to list. It is estimated that there could be as many as 100 million different species on Earth, although nowhere near that many have been physically catalogued. Of these, the majority are Bacteria and Archaea.

Another Example - Homo Sapiens

Since there is no way to list all of the different subdivisions of life on Earth here, we might as well focus on one specific animal: us, Homo sapiens. We are members of the Domain Eukarya, the Kingdom Animalia, the Phylum Chordata, the Class Mammalia, the Order Primates, the Family Hominidae, the Genus Homo, the Species Homo sapiens and finally the Subspecies Homo sapiens sapiens. This classification is able to demonstrate our exact biological position in relation to life on Earth.

One important thing a system like this tells us is that Homo, which is Latin for "human," is not actually our species, but our genus. This is an easy fact to forget since we are currently the only member of our genus not yet extinct. But anthropologically speaking there have been many humans including Homo habilis, Homo erectus and Homo neanderthalensis.

Taxonomical classification is an evolutionary map

Furthermore, the taxonomical classification system can be seen as a map of evolution on the planet. Plants, animals and bacteria can be traced back to common ancestors and newly discovered species can be classified in relation to their ancestors, descendants and cousins. The Genus Homo, for instance, is a direct offshoot of the Tribe Hominini. (A tribe is a subcategory of the category of family, which in this case is Hominidae.) Another genus that falls under the Tribe Hominini is Pan, which houses the species Chimpanzee. This shows us that until relatively recently in the history of life, Homo sapiens and Chimpanzees were the same creature, and that Chimpanzees only split off just before Homo sapiens became fully human.

Chemistry

Chemistry is the science of matter, especially its chemical reactions, but also its composition, structure and properties. Chemistry is concerned with atoms and their interactions with other atoms, and particularly with the properties of chemical bonds.

Chemistry is sometimes called "the central science" because it connects physics with other natural sciences such as geology and biology. Chemistry is a branch of physical science but distinct from physics.

Traditional chemistry starts with the study of elementary particles, atoms, molecules, substances, metals, crystals and other aggregates of matter. in solid, liquid, and gas states, whether in isolation or combination. The interactions, reactions and transformations that are studied in chemistry are a result of interaction either between different chemical substances or between matter and energy.

A chemical reaction is a transformation of some substances into one or more other substances.

It can be symbolically depicted through a chemical equation. The number of atoms on the left and the right in the equation for a chemical transformation is most often equal. The nature of chemical reactions a substance may undergo and the energy changes that may accompany it are constrained by certain basic rules, known as chemical laws.

Energy and entropy considerations are invariably important in almost all chemical studies.

Chemical substances are classified in terms of their structure, phase as well as their chemical compositions. They can be analyzed using the tools of chemical analysis, e.g. spectroscopy and chromatography. Scientists engaged in chemical research are known as chemists. Most chemists specialize in one or more sub-disciplines. [8]

Basic Concepts in Chemistry

Atoms

Atoms are some of the basic building blocks of matter. Each atom is an element—an identifiable substance that cannot be further broken down into other identifiable substances.

There are just over 100 such elements, and each of them can combine with themselves and with other elements to create all the various molecules that exist in the universe. The poison gas chlorine and the explosive metal sodium, for instance, can combine at the atomic level to form sodium chloride, also known as salt.

For thousands of years atoms were thought to be the smallest thing possible. (The word "atom" comes from an ancient Greek word meaning "unbreakable.") However, experiments performed in the mid to late 19th century began to show the presence of small particles, electrons, in electric current. By the early 20th century, the electron was known to be a part of the atom that orbited a yet undefined atomic core. A few years later, in 1919, the proton was discovered and found to exist in the nuclei of all atoms.

The protons and neutrons inside an atomic nucleus are not fundamental particles. That is, they can be divided into still smaller pieces.

Protons and neutrons are known as hadrons, which is a class of particle made up of quarks. (Quarks are a fundamental particle.) There are two distinct types of hadrons, baryons and mesons, and both protons and neutrons are baryons, meaning they are both made up of a combination of three quarks. In addition to being hadrons, protons and neutrons are also known as nucleons because of their place within the nucleus. Protons have a mass of around $1.6726 \times 10{-27}$ kg and neutrons have a nearly identical mass of $1.6929 \times 10{-27}$ kg. Both particles have a ½ spin.

The number of protons inside an atomic nucleus determines what element the atom is.

An element with only one proton, for instance, is hydrogen. An element with two is helium. One with three is lithium, and so on. No element (with the exception of hydrogen) can exist with only protons in its nucleus. Atoms need neutrons to bond the protons together using the strong force. In general atoms (again except for hydrogen) have an equal number of protons and neutrons in their nuclei.

Atoms with an uneven number of protons and neutrons are called isotopes.

Isotopes have all the same chemical properties as their evenly balanced counterparts, but their nuclei are not usually as stable and are more willing to react with other elements. (Two deuterium atoms, hydrogen isotopes with one proton and one neutron in their nucleus rather than only one proton, will fuse much more readily than two regular hydrogen atoms.)

Nearly all of an atoms' mass is within its nucleus. Outside of that there is a lot of empty space occupied only by a few, tiny electrons.

Electrons were once viewed as orbiting an atom like planets orbit the sun. We now know that this is wrong in several ways. For one, electrons do not really "orbit" in the sense we are used to. At the quantum level no particle is really a particle, but is actually both a particle and a wave simultaneously. Heisenberg's uncertainty principle looks at this odd truth about reality and says that at no time can you watch an electron orbit the nucleus as you would watch the Earth orbit the sun. Instead, you have to observe only one of the electron's physical characteristics at a time, either viewing it as a particle in a fixed position outside the nucleus or as a wave encircling the nucleus like a halo.
Additionally, planets orbiting their stars can orbit at any distance they want. In fact, every object in our solar system has an elliptical orbit, meaning that they all move in more oval rather than circular shapes, getting closer and farther from the sun at various points. Electrons cannot do this under any circumstances.

Atoms have what are known as electron shells, which are the levels that an electron is able to occupy.

Electrons cannot exist in between these shells; instead they jump from one to the next instantaneously. Each electron shell can hold a different number of atoms. When a shell fills up, additional electrons fill the outer shells. The outermost shell of any atom is called the valence shell, and it is the electrons in this shell that interact with the electrons of other atoms. The important thing about the valence shell is that each electron shell has a specific number of electrons that it can hold, and it wants to hold that many.

When atoms join together; their connecting valence electrons take up two valence shell spots, one on each atom.

This means that the fewer electrons an atom has in its valence shell, the more likely it is to interact with other atoms. Conversely, the more electrons it has, the less likely it is to interact.

Electrons can also momentarily jump from one electron shell to the next if they are hit with a burst of energy from a photon.

When photons hit atoms, the energy is briefly absorbed by the electrons, and this momentarily knocks them into higher "orbits." The particular "orbit" the electron is knocked into depends on the type of atom, and when the electron gives up its higher energy level it re-emits a photon at a slightly different wavelength than the one it absorbed, providing a characteristic signal of that atom and showing exactly what "orbit" the electron was knocked into.

This is the phenomenon responsible for spectral lines in light and is the reason we can tell what elements make up stars and planets just by looking at them.

Unlike protons and neutrons, electrons are a fundamental particle all on their own. They are known as leptons.

Electrons have a negative charge that is generally balanced out by the positive charge of their atom's protons.

Charged atoms, which have either gained or lost an electron for various reasons, are called ions.

Ions, like isotopes, have the same properties that the regular element does; they simply have different tendencies towards reacting with other atoms. Electrons have a mass of $9.1094 \times 10\text{-}31$ kg and a -½ spin.

Element

The concept of chemical element is related to that of chemical substance. A chemical element is specifically a substance which is composed of a single type of atom.

A chemical element is characterized by a particular number of protons in the nuclei of its atoms. This number is known as the atomic number of the element. For example, all atoms with 6 protons in their nuclei are atoms of the chemical element carbon, and all atoms with 92 protons in their nuclei are atoms of the element uranium.

Compound

A compound is a substance with a particular ratio of atoms of particular chemical elements which determines its composition, and a particular organization which determines chemical properties.

For example, water is a compound containing hydrogen and oxygen in the ratio of two to one, with the oxygen atom between the two hydrogen atoms, and an angle of 104.5° between them. Compounds are formed and interconverted by chemical reactions.

Substance

A chemical substance is a kind of matter with a definite composition and set of properties.

Strictly speaking, a mixture of compounds, elements or compounds and elements is not a chemical substance, but it may be called a chemical. Most of the substances we encounter in our daily life are some kind of mixture; for example: air, alloys, biomass, etc.

Nomenclature of substances is a critical part of the language of chemistry. Generally it refers to a system for naming chemical compounds.

Earlier in the history of chemistry substances were given names by their discoverer, which often led to some confusion and difficulty. However, today the IUPAC system of chemical nomenclature allows chemists to specify by name specific compounds amongst the vast variety of possible chemicals.

The standard nomenclature of chemical substances is set by the International Union of Pure and Applied Chemistry (IUPAC). There are well-defined systems in place for naming chemical species. Organic compounds are named according to the organic nomenclature system. Inorganic compounds are named according to the inorganic nomenclature system. In addition the Chemical Abstracts Service has devised a method to index chemical substance. In this scheme each chemical substance is identifiable by a number known as CAS registry number.

Molecule

Molecules are two or more atoms joined together through a chemical bond to form chemicals.

Molecules differ from atoms in that molecules can be further broken down into smaller pieces and into elements while atoms cannot. (This was actually the 18th century definition of an atom: a recognizable structure that could no longer be broken down into smaller bits.)

Atoms are joined together into molecules in two main ways: through covalent bonds and through ionic bonds.

Covalent bonds are the primary type of chemical bond that forms molecules. They occur when atoms with only partially filled valence electron shells, an atom's outermost electron shell, come together to share electrons. Hydrogen atoms, for instance, each have only one electron, while their valence shell is capable of holding two. When two hydrogen atoms come together each share the other's electron, using it to occupy its valence shell's free space forming the H2 molecule: hydrogen gas.

Not all covalent bond's are the same.

Different atoms have different levels of positive charge coming from in their nuclei, and although, under normal circumstances, the negative charge of the atom's electrons balances that out (keeping the atom electrically neutral) the chemical bonding process has a way of exploiting this situation. If we look at the H2 molecule again, everyday experience tells us that it has a strong tendency to seek out and bond with oxygen (O) molecules forming H20, or water. There are two main reasons for this. The first comes from the regular old covalent bonds that are already holding H2 together. If bonded to another atom, hydrogen gains the ability to form a new valence shell that can hold 6 electrons. Since oxygen is the only molecule to naturally have 6 electrons in its valence shell, it is the most eager to bond with hydrogen. However, oxygen also has 8 protons in its nucleus compared to the total of 2 in the H2 molecule. This means that as the atoms come closer and prepare to bond, the electrons from both atoms are pulled closer to the oxygen molecule and farther from the hydrogen. An atom's proclivity to pull electrons towards itself is called its electronegativity, and this process creates polar covalent bonds. Due to this connection, polar covalent bonds are the strongest molecular bond, which is why molecules like water are so prevalent in our solar system and, likely, throughout the galaxy.

One very interesting aspect of polar covalent bonds is the hydrogen bond.

When a hydrogen atom bonds with another electronegative atom, the newly created molecule develops an intense polar attraction to all other electronegative atoms. This attraction works almost like a magnet with one end of the molecule exhibiting a positive charge (due to the effects of the polar covalent bonds pulling all of the electrons towards one end of the molecule) and the other end exhibiting a negative charge. This phenomenon is responsible for, among other things, the way water molecules stick to each other so readily. This is why you can fill a glass of water to a millimeter or so above the rim before it spills.

Hydrogen bonds are also responsible for how hydrophilic and hydrophobic molecules react to being mixed with water.

Hydrophilic molecules are molecules like NaCl (salt) which exhibit their own strong charge for reasons we will discuss in a moment. The charged salt molecules mix eagerly with the charged water molecules due to the extra pull of the hydrogen bond. Conversely, hydrophobic molecules such as oil will not mix with water because they are neutrally charged and do not like charged molecules. This is the reason you have to shake up an oil based salad dressing each time you use it. The oil and the water never truly mix, and given only a short amount of time they will separate.

A very different type of bond between atoms is called the ionic bond.

Ionic bonds only occur between ions, atoms that are either positively or negatively charged due to having an unequal number of protons and electrons. Ionic bonds always occur between metals and non-metals, such as the gas chlorine (Cl) and the alkaline metal sodium (Na). In their normal states, neither of these elements are ions, but when they approach each other, the sodium gives the chlorine one of its electrons forming Cl- and Na+ ions, which subsequently become attracted to one another. Since no electrons are actually lost, the molecule still technically has a neutral charge; it is only the atoms that are charged.

In ionic bonds it is always the metal which gives its electron to the non-metal. Additionally, in a diluted or liquid form, molecules that are created like this will always conduct electricity. This is why salt water can make such a good conductor.

Ions and salts

An ion is a charged species, an atom or a molecule, that has lost or gained one or more electrons.

Positively charged cations (e.g. sodium cation $Na+$) and negatively charged anions (e.g. chloride $Cl-$) can form a crystalline lattice of neutral salts (e.g. sodium chloride $NaCl$). Examples of polyatomic ions that do not split up during acid-base reactions are hydroxide ($OH-$) and phosphate ($PO43-$).

Ions in the gaseous phase are often known as plasma.

Acidity and basicity

A substance can often be classified as an acid or a base. There are several different theories which explain acid-base behavior. The simplest is Arrhenius theory.

The Arrhenius theory states than an acid is a substance that produces hydronium ions when it is dissolved in water, and a base is one that produces hydroxide ions when dissolved in water. According to Brønsted–Lowry acid-base theory, acids are substances that donate a positive hydrogen ion to another substance in a chemical reaction; by extension, a base is the substance which receives that hydrogen ion.

A third common theory is Lewis acid-base theory, which is based on the formation of new chemical bonds.

Lewis theory explains that an acid is a substance which is capable of accepting a pair of electrons from another substance during the process of bond formation, while a base is a substance which can provide a pair of electrons to form a new bond. According to concept as per Lewis, the crucial things being exchanged are charges. There are several other ways in which a substance may be classified as an acid or a base, as is evident in the history of this concept

Acid strength is commonly measured by two methods. The most common is pH.

One measurement, based on the Arrhenius definition of acidity, is pH, which is a measurement of the hydronium ion concentration in a solution, as expressed on a negative logarithmic scale. Thus, solutions that have a low pH have a high hydronium ion concentration, and can be said to be more acidic. The other measurement, based on the Brønsted–Lowry definition, is the acid dissociation constant (Ka), which measure the relative ability of a substance to act as an acid under the Brønsted–Lowry definition of an acid. That is, substances with a higher Ka are more likely to donate hydrogen ions in chemical reactions than those with lower Ka values.

Phase

In addition to the specific chemical properties that distinguish chemical classifications, chemicals can exist in several phases.

For the most part, the chemical classifications are independent of these bulk phase classifications; however, some more exotic phases are incompatible with certain chemical properties. A phase is a set of states of a chemical system that have similar bulk structural properties, over a range of conditions, such as pressure or temperature.

Physical properties, such as density and refractive index tend to fall within values characteristic of the phase. The phase of matter is defined by the phase transition, which is when energy put into or taken out of the system goes into rearranging the structure of the system, instead of changing the bulk conditions.

Phase can be continuous.

Sometimes the distinction between phases can be continuous instead of having a discrete boundary, in this case the matter is considered to be in a supercritical state. When three states meet based on the conditions, it is known as a triple point and since this is invariant, it is a convenient way to define a set of conditions.

The most familiar examples of phases are solids, liquids, and gases. Many substances exhibit multiple solid phases. For example, there are three phases of solid iron (alpha, gamma, and delta) that vary based on temperature and pressure. A principal difference between solid phases is the crystal structure, or arrangement, of the atoms. Another phase commonly encountered in the study of chemistry is the aqueous phase, which is the state of substances dissolved in aqueous solution (that is, in water).

Less familiar phases include plasmas, Bose-Einstein condensates and fermionic condensates and the paramagnetic and ferromagnetic phases of magnetic materials. While most familiar phases deal with three-dimensional systems, it is also possible to define analogs in two-dimensional systems, which has received attention for its relevance to systems in biology.

Redox

Redox is a concept related to the ability of atoms of various substances to lose or gain electrons.

Substances that have the ability to oxidize other substances are said to be oxidative and are known as oxidizing agents, oxidants or oxidizers. An oxidant removes electrons from another substance. Similarly, substances that have the ability to reduce other substances are said to be reductive and are known as reducing agents, reductants, or reducers.

A reductant transfers electrons to another substance, and is thus oxidized itself. And because it "donates" electrons it is also called an electron donor.

Oxidation and reduction properly refer to a change in oxidation number—the actual transfer of electrons may never occur. Thus, oxidation is better defined as an increase in oxidation number, and reduction as a decrease in oxidation number.

Bonding

Electron atomic and molecular orbitals

Atoms sticking together in molecules or crystals are said to be bonded with one another.

A chemical bond may be visualized as the multipole balance between the positive charges in the nuclei and the negative charges oscillating about them. More than simple attraction and repulsion, the energies and distributions characterize the availability of an electron to bond to another atom.

A chemical bond can be a covalent bond, an ionic bond, a hydrogen bond or just because of Van der Waals force.

Each of these kinds of bond is ascribed to some potential. These potentials create the interactions which hold atoms together in molecules or crystals. In many simple compounds, Valence Bond Theory, the Valence Shell Electron Pair Repulsion model (VSEPR), and the concept of oxidation number can be used to explain molecular structure and composition.

Reaction

During chemical reactions, bonds between atoms break and form, resulting in different substances with different properties.

In a blast furnace, iron oxide, a compound, reacts with carbon monoxide to form iron, one of the chemical elements, and carbon dioxide.

When a chemical substance is transformed as a result of its interaction with another or energy, a chemical reaction is said to have occurred. Chemical reaction is therefore a concept related to the 'reaction' of a substance when it comes in close contact with another, whether as a mixture or a solution; exposure to some form of energy, or both. It results in some energy exchange between the constituents of the reaction as well with the system environment which may be designed vessels which are often laboratory glassware.

Chemical reactions can result in the formation or dissociation of molecules, that is, molecules breaking apart to form two or more smaller molecules, or rearrangement of atoms within or across molecules.

Chemical reactions usually involve the making or breaking of chemical bonds. Oxidation, reduction, dissociation, acid-base neutralization and molecular rearrangement are some of the commonly used kinds of chemical reactions.

A chemical reaction can be symbolically depicted through a chemical equation. While in a non-nuclear chemical reaction the number and kind of atoms on both sides of the equation are equal, for a nuclear reaction this holds true only for the nuclear particles viz. protons and neutrons.

The sequence of steps in which the reorganization of chemical bonds may be taking place in the course of a chemical reaction is called its mechanism.

A chemical reaction can be envisioned to take place in a number of steps, each of which may have a different speed. Many reaction intermediates with variable stability can thus be envisaged during the course of a reaction. Reaction mechanisms are proposed to explain the kinetics and the relative product mix of a reaction. Many physical chemists specialize in exploring and proposing the mechanisms of various chemical reactions. Several empirical rules, like the Woodward-Hoffmann rules often come handy while proposing a mechanism for a chemical reaction.

Equilibrium

Although the concept of equilibrium is widely used across sciences, in the context of chemistry, it arises whenever a number of different states of the chemical composition are possible.

For example, in a mixture of several chemical compounds that can react with one another, or when a substance can be present in more than one kind of phase.

A system of chemical substances at equilibrium even though having an unchanging composition is most often not static; molecules of the substances continue to react with one another thus giving rise to a dynamic equilibrium. Thus the concept describes the state in which the parameters such as chemical composition remain unchanged over time. Chemicals present in biological systems are invariably not at equilibrium; rather they are far from equilibrium.

The Periodic Table

The periodic table contains the known chemical elements displayed in a special tabular arrangement based on their electron configurations, atomic numbers and recurring chemical properties.

The first semblance of a periodic table was by Antoine Lavoisier in 1789. He published a list or table of the 33 chemical elements known as of that time. He grouped the elements into earths, non-metals, gases and metals. The next century after that discovery saw several chemists looking for a better classification method and this gave rise to the periodic table as we have it today.

Structure of the Periodic Table

The standard periodic table as it is today is an 18 column by 7 rows table containing the main chemical elements. Beneath that is a smaller 15 column by 2 rows table. The periodic table can be broken down into 4 rectangular blocks: the P block is by the right, S block is left, D block is at the middle and the F block is underneath that. The elements in the blocks are based on which sub-shell the last electron resides.

The chemical elements on the table are arranged in order of increasing atomic number, which refers to the number of protons of the element. The periodic table can be used to study the chemical behavior of chemical elements, which makes it a very important tool widely used in chemistry.

The periodic table contains only chemical elements. Mixtures, compounds or small atomic particles of elements are not included. Each element on the table has a unique atomic number, which represents the number of protons contained in the element's nucleus.

A new period or row begins when an element has a new electron shell with a first electron. Columns or groups are based on the configuration of electrons of the atom. Elements that have an equal number of atoms in a specific sub-shell are listed under the same column. For example, selenium and oxygen both have 4 electrons in their outermost sub shell and so are listed under the P column. Elements with similar properties are listed in the same group although some elements in the same period can also share similar properties too. Since the elements grouped together have related properties, one can easily predict the property of an element if the properties of the surrounding elements are already known.

Rows are Periods

The rows of the periodic table are referred to as periods. Elements on a row have the same number of electron shells or atomic orbitals. Elements on the first row have just one atomic orbital, elements on the second row have 2, and so it goes until the elements on the seventh row have 7 electron shells or atomic orbitals.

Columns are Groups

Columns from up to down in the table are called groups. The columns in the D, P and S blocks are referred to as groups. Elements within a group have equal number of electrons in their outermost electron shell or orbital. The electrons on the outer shell are called valence electrons and there are the electrons that combine with other elements in a chemical reaction.

The Periodic table contains natural and synthesized elements

The elements up to californium are natural existing elements (94) while the rest were laboratory synthesized. Till date, chemists are still working to produce elements beyond the present 118th element, ununoctium. 114 of the 118 elements on the table have been officially recognized by the International Union of Pure and Applied Chemistry (IUPAC). Elements listed on the table under 113, 115, 117 and 118 have been synthesized but are yet to officially recognized by the IUPAC and are only known by their systematic element names.

Group → Period ↓	1	2	3	4	5	6	7	8	9	10	11	12	13	14	15	16	17	18
1	1 H																	2 He
2	3 Li	4 Be											5 B	6 C	7 N	8 O	9 F	10 Ne
3	11 Na	12 Mg											13 Al	14 Si	15 P	16 S	17 Cl	18 Ar
4	19 K	20 Ca	21 Sc	22 Ti	23 V	24 Cr	25 Mn	26 Fe	27 Co	28 Ni	29 Cu	30 Zn	31 Ga	32 Ge	33 As	34 Se	35 Br	36 Kr
5	37 Rb	38 Sr	39 Y	40 Zr	41 Nb	42 Mo	43 Tc	44 Ru	45 Rh	46 Pd	47 Ag	48 Cd	49 In	50 Sn	51 Sb	52 Te	53 I	54 Xe
6	55 Cs	56 Ba		72 Hf	73 Ta	74 W	75 Re	76 Os	77 Ir	78 Pt	79 Au	80 Hg	81 Tl	82 Pb	83 Bi	84 Po	85 At	86 Rn
7	87 Fr	88 Ra		104 Rf	105 Db	106 Sg	107 Bh	108 Hs	109 Mt	110 Ds	111 Rg	112 Cn	113 Uut	114 Fl	115 Uup	116 Lv	117 Uus	118 Uuo

Lanthanides	57 La	58 Ce	59 Pr	60 Nd	61 Pm	62 Sm	63 Eu	64 Gd	65 Tb	66 Dy	67 Ho	68 Er	69 Tm	70 Yb	71 Lu
Actinides	89 Ac	90 Th	91 Pa	92 U	93 Np	94 Pu	95 Am	96 Cm	97 Bk	98 Cf	99 Es	100 Fm	101 Md	102 No	103 Lr

Basic Physics

Kinetic and Mechanical Energy

The kinetic energy of an object is the energy it possesses due to its motion.

Kinetic energy is defined as the work needed to accelerate a body of a given mass from rest to a stated velocity. Like all forms of energy, kinetic energy is measured in joules. Kinetic energy can be imparted to an object when an energy source is tapped to accelerate it. It can also happen when one object with kinetic energy slams into another object and kinetic energy from the first object is transferred to the second.

However it happens, imparting kinetic energy to an object causes it to accelerate. In this way movement is nothing more than an indication of the amount of kinetic energy an object has. An object will hold onto its kinetic energy until it is able to transfer it to something else, which allows it to slow down again.

As long as an object has the same level of kinetic energy, it will move at a consistent velocity forever. This is Newton's first law of motion.

The transfer of kinetic energy from one object to another can occur in many ways.

The transfer of kinetic energy can be as simple and mundane as a baseball flying through the air—interacting with all the various molecules of oxygen, carbon dioxide, nitrogen and all the other gasses that make up our atmosphere, and transferring its kinetic energy to them—speeding them up and slowing itself down in the process. Or it can be as chaotic as a speeding truck losing control on an icy road and slamming into a wall.

Different types of interactions between objects appear to be different but are in fact the same.

The interaction between the baseball and the air and between the truck and the wall are only superficially different. One appears more chaotic than the other only because of the differences in mass between a baseball and a truck and the differences in "negative energy" possessed by free-floating air molecules compared to a solid wall. At its most basic, however, the same events are taking place in both examples. Molecules in the both wall and the air scatter when the kinetic energy they receive causes them to move, and this causes both heat and sound to be produced.

Kinetic energy can be calculated with the formula $KE=\frac{1}{2}mv^2$ where m is the mass of the object in kilograms, and v is its velocity in meters/second.

Kinetic energy increases by the square of an objects velocity.

One important aspect of kinetic energy that makes it so potentially destructive is that the kinetic energy a moving object carries does not increase on pace with its velocity, but rather in relation to the square of its velocity. If you double an object's velocity, you will quadruple the amount of kinetic energy it possesses (22=4). If you quadruple the velocity, you increase the kinetic energy by sixteen times (42=16). This can lead to relatively small masses possessing very high kinetic energy levels when they are accelerated to only nominally high speeds. This is one reason why modern kinetic energy weapons (such as firearms) are able to cause large amounts of damage while being extremely compact.

Mechanical Energy

Mechanical energy is the ability of an object to do work.

When discussing energy it is important to take a moment to understand mechanical energy and how it relates to the objects it interacts with. Mechanical energy is not a separate type of energy in the way that potential energy and kinetic energy differ from each other.

Mechanical energy is the potential energy available to an object added to all of the kinetic energy available to it, providing a total energy output.

For instance, in our description of potential energy there is the example of a pole-vaulter hanging in mid-air with her pole bent at a near right angle to the ground. The bend in the pole-vaulter's pole contains elastic potential energy, which will help her clear the bar. However, that is not the only source of energy the pole-vaulter is restricted to. For anyone who has ever seen a track and field competition, you know that pole-vaulters take long, running starts before planting their poles in the ground. This imparts kinetic energy to the runners body, and it is that kinetic energy plus the pole's elastic potential energy that are added together in mid-air to impart the total mechanical energy that drives the pole-vaulter high into the air and over the bar.

Potential Energy

There are two main types of potential energy: gravitational potential energy and elastic potential energy.

Potential energy is quite simply the potential an object has to act on other objects. In the form of gravitational potential energy, the object is raised off the ground and is waiting for the force of gravity pulling at $9.8 m/s^2$, to grab hold of it and pull it towards the Earth.

This type of energy is very common in everyday life. It describes everything from a book falling off its shelf to a child tripping on a crack in the sidewalk. Because gravitational potential energy is so common, the equation describing it PEgrav=mass*g*height should not be hard to figure out since it contains only easily observable features of matter: an object's mass, the force of gravity (g), and the object's height off the ground when it started falling.

Note that the height does not have to be measured from the ground. Any point can be chosen—such as a table top or even a point in mid-air—provided that you are only concerned with the energy an object would have if it fell from the point it was currently at to the point you have chosen.

Gravitational Potential Energy Example

If we take the example of a 1kg weight positioned at a height of 1 meter above the surface of Earth (where the gravity is $9.8 m/s^2$—try this on Mars and you will get a different result), we end up with the equation PEgrav=1*9.8*1, which equals 9.8 joules of gravitational potential energy. A 1g weight positioned at the same height would be PEgrav=.001*9.8*1 or .0098J of potential energy, while a 1kg weight positioned a kilometer up would equal PEgrav=1*9.8*1000 or 9800J of potential energy.

From this equation you may have picked up on the fact that the height an object is raised to is directly proportional to the amount of gravitational potential energy it has. Take a 1kg object and raise it to 5m, and you get 49J of potential energy. Double that to 10m, and you get 98J. Triple it to 15m and you will get 147J—three times the original 49J.

Elastic Potential Energy

Elastic potential energy occurs when an object is stretched or compressed out of its normal "resting" shape. The amount of energy that will be released when it finally returns to rest is the amount of elastic potential energy it has while stretched or compressed.

A common example of elastic potential energy is when an archer draws back the string of his bow. The farther back the bowstring is pulled, the more it will stretch. The more it stretches the more potential energy it will have waiting to send into the arrow.

Elastic potential energy of an object can be determined using Hooke's law of elasticity. Hooke's law states that F=-kx where F is the force the material will exert as it returns to its resting state measured in Newtons, x is amount of displacement the material undergoes measured in meters, and k is the spring constant and is measured in Newtons/meter.

In order to determine the potential energy of an elastic or springy material you use the equation PE = $1/2\ kx^2$. According to this equation, an object such as a spring with a spring constant of 5N/m that is stretched 3 meters past its resting point would have a potential energy of 22.5J. That is, 1/2 * 5 * 32 = 2.5 * 9 = 22.5J.
Remember that elastic potential energy affects much more than just what you would consider elastic or springy material such as rubber bands, bungee cords and springs. There is elastic potential energy in a pole-vaulter's pole at the point where she is in the air and hanging onto a pole that is bent nearly sideways. In the next instant her forward momentum will be boosted by the conversion of her pole's potential energy into kinetic energy, pushing her over the bar. Similarly, when a hockey player shoots the puck, he drags his stick along the ice as it moves forward, bending the shaft backwards slightly. This adds extra force to the puck as the stick snaps forward back into its normal resting position.

Energy: Work and Power

In the simplest terms, energy is the ability to do work.

Energy allows objects and people to affect the physical world and displace (or move) other objects or people.

Work in the physics sense is a very specific concept.

It is measured in joules, which are defined as being 1 Newton of force that displaces something by 1 meter. (J=Nm) As the mass of the object being displaced varies, the amount of work in joules required to move it a meter will vary too.

To determine the amount of work being done, you can use the equation W=F*d*cosΘ.

This defines work as the force applied, multiplied by the distance the object was displaced, multiplied by the cosine of Θ (Theta).

The force is measured in Newtons. Distance is measured in meters. The tricky part of this equation is determining the cosine of Θ. Θ represents the difference in angle between the vector (or direction) the force is acting in and the vector the displacement is occurring. That means that there are really only three possible values for Θ.

If the force is pushing or pulling in one direction, and the object being displaced is moving in that same direction, then there is no difference in angle between the vectors and Θ=0°. This is the sort of force you get when a child pulls her sled across a snowy field. The direction the child is pulling and the direction the sled is traveling are the same. Since cos0=1 the amount of work is determined simply by multiplying the force and the displacement.

You should note that the angle of the vectors is determined by their relationship to each other and not to some sort of ideal flat surface. That is, if the child is pulling her sled up a steep hill rather than across a field, the angle of Θ is still going to be 0° since the force she exerts on the sled and the sled itself are still traveling in the same direction.

The second possibility is when the force vector acts in the opposite direction of the object's displacement. This gives you what is called "negative work" because the energy is working to hinder the object from moving rather than to help it. In this instance Θ=180° since the vector in which the force is acting and the vector in which the object is moving are opposite. This force is most commonly observed when dealing with friction. It is the reason that hockey pucks and soccer balls will not travel forever; the force of friction exerted by the ice and by the grass is acting in the opposite direction.

The final difference in vectors is when the force being exerted on an object is at a right angle to its displacement. In this case Θ=90°. You can picture this as a waitress carrying a tray of drinks over to your table, and it provides for some odd conclusions. Since the force we are talking about is the force the waitress is using to hold the tray vertically, but the displacement vector of the tray is horizontally across the room, we find that the force the waitress exerts does no work at all. It is not responsible for moving the tray horizontally towards your table.

This is represented mathematically with the fact that the cos90=0, meaning that the original equation W=F*d*cosΘ would be W=F*d*0. Without adding any other information in, it is already obvious that work is going to equal zero joules.

A different way to imagine this is to think of cargo in the back of a truck.

It took work to load the cargo up onto the truck from the ground (the force vector and the displacement vector were both pointing in the same direction), but once the cargo was loaded, no additional work was required to keep it there. The truck could drive from one end of the country to the other, but zero joules of work would be exerted keeping the cargo in place in the back of the truck.

When you add a unit of time to your calculations of work, you get a new classification: power.

Power is the rate at which work is done. The equation that measures power is power=work/time. In this equation work is measured in joules, time is measured in seconds and power is measured in watts.
Since, as we noted above, one joule is the same as one Newton multiplied by one meter, this equation can also be written as power=(force*displacement)/time where force is measured in Newtons and displacement is measured in meters. But, this opens up further possibilities. Since the math does not care whether we first multiply force with displacement before dividing the whole thing by time, or whether we divide displacement by time and then multiply the answer by force, we find the equation can also be written as power=force(displacement/time).

Given that displacement is measured in meters and the time in seconds, what we are really saying here is that power equals the amount of force applied to an object multiplied by that object's velocity (m/s).

Thus we get two equations describing power: power=work/time and power=force*velocity.

By definition, power has an inverse relationship with time; the less time it takes for the work to be done, the more power is being applied. Power also has a direct relationship with force and velocity. Increase either the amount of force being applied to an object, or the speed at which it is traveling, and you have increased the power.

Defining Force and Newton's Three Laws

In physics force is the term given to anything that has the power to act on an object, causing its displacement in one direction or another.

Forces are a somewhat abstract concept, and it is for that reason that it took thousands of years to accurately identify and describe them. It was not until the 17th century when a man named Isaac Newton began to accurately describe the basic physical forces and show how they acted on matter.

Force is measured using the unit Newton (N). One Newton can be defined with the formula $1N=1kg(1m/s^2)$. In other words, if you accelerate a kilogram of matter by one meter per second per second, you have exerted one Newton of force on it.

Newton developed three laws to explain the interactions of matter he observed. The first is often known as the "Law of Inertia."

It states that an object at rest will stay at rest, and an object in motion will stay in motion, unless a force acts upon it to change its state. This means that if you fire a spaceship out into the vacuum of space, and keep it clear from planets and stars that will apply force to it, the ship will keep going at the same speed forever.

This tendency to stay moving or stay at rest is known as inertia. Inertia is directly related to an object's mass; the more mass an object has, the more inertia it will have and the harder it will be to speed it up or slow it down. This is implied by the equation defining one Newton of force, but it is also obvious in everyday life. You have to exert more force to push a box of books across the floor than you would to push a box of clothes the same size. The box of books has more mass, so it has more inertia. Similarly, a baseball player can easily catch and stop a baseball thrown at over 100km/hr. If you were to ask that same player to stop a truck traveling at 100km/hr, you would get much less pleasant results.

One important thing to remember about force is that it is a vector quantity, meaning that it points in a specific direction.

Set a one kilogram object down on a table and you will have the force of gravity pulling it down at one Newton, and the force of all the atoms in the table pushing it up at one Newton. This is said to be a state of equilibrium, and it causes no change to the object's velocity. However, if the table had been poorly built and was only capable of pushing up at .75 Newtons, the object would pull through, snapping the table at its weakest points, and fall until it found something that was capable of applying the needed force to hold it up against gravity.

As such, an object can only be at rest if it has no forces acting on it, or if it has equal and opposite forces acting on it keeping it at equilibrium. If an unopposed force acts on an object, it will move.

Newton's second law deals with what happens when you have the sort of unbalanced forces that we just described.

It explains the movement of objects through the equation $F=ma$, where F is the force in Newtons, m is the object's mass in kilograms, and a is the object's acceleration in meters per second per second (m/s2).

Just like with Newton's first law, this equation shows that mass is a huge player when it comes to using a force to move objects. The larger the mass, the more force you will need to accelerate or decelerate it to the same velocity.

Newton's third law states simply that for every action there is an equal and opposite reaction.

This means that if I pound my hand down on my desk right now, my desk will also be hitting up at my hand with the exact same force. This may sound strange, but it is the reason that pounding your hand on your desk can damage your desk and hurt your hand at the same time. It is also the reason that baseball bats can snap while imparting force onto the ball, and why a moving car hitting stationary wall will damage both.

Force: Friction

Friction is the force that resists the motion of objects in relation to other objects.

When two surfaces move in relation to each other, the force of friction is what slows them down. Friction applies to all matter, whether it is a book sliding down a slanting shelf, a soccer ball rolling on the ground or a baseball flying though the air. Essentially, friction is a constant opposing force that keeps things from traveling forever.

Several laws describe how friction works.

Amontons' first law of friction says that, "The force of friction is directly proportional to the applied load." His second law of friction says that, "The force of friction is independent of the apparent area of contact." Similarly, Coulomb's law of friction states that, "Kinetic friction is independent of the sliding velocity."

The two main types of Friction are static friction and kinetic friction.

Static friction is what you get when one stationary object is stacked on top of another stationary object, such as a book resting on a table. The static friction between the book and the table determines how much sticking power there is between them, and at what angle you would have to tilt the table before the force of gravity overpowers the force of friction and starts the book sliding.

To figure out the maximum amount of static friction possible before the book starts sliding, you use the formula $f_s = \mu_s F_n$ where f_s is the total amount of static friction, μ_s (pronounced "mu") is the coefficient of static friction and F_n is the "normal force," the force being exerted perpendicularly through the surface into the object resting on it, keeping the object from breaking through the surface.

Another way to examine static friction is to calculate the angle the table will have to reach before the book will start sliding.

This is also known as the angle of repose, and it can be calculated using the formula $\tan\theta=\mu s$ where θ (pronounced "theta") is the angle of repose and μs is the coefficient of static friction.

Aside from determining the angels that books will slide off tables, calculating static friction allows tire manufacturers to determine how "grippy" their treads are. If there were no friction, the wheel would not be a functional tool because it would not push itself against the road while moving. The higher the coefficient of friction between the tire and the road, the more grip the tire has.

Kinetic friction is sort of the inverse of static friction.

It is the force that causes moving objects to slow down. Kinetic friction applies to two surfaces moving in respect to one another such as the bottom of a snowboard and the snowy ground. It can be calculated using the same basic formula used to calculate static friction: $fk=\mu kFn$ with the only differences being the sub-k marks replacing the sub-s marks of the previous equation, signifying kinetic friction.

As kinetic friction slows an object, the object's kinetic energy is transformed into heat.

Fundamental Forces: Electromagnetism

Electromagnetism is one of the four fundamental forces. It is far more common than gravity, but only if you know where to look.

Electromagnetism is responsible for nearly all interactions in which gravity plays no part. It is what holds negatively charged electrons in orbit around the positively charged protons in the nucleus of an atom. It is also the force that joins atoms to each other to create molecules.

It is also electromagnetism that is responsible for the fact that matter—which is made up of atoms and at the subatomic level is mostly empty space—feels solid.

When you sit down in your chair, it is the electromagnetic attraction between the chair's atoms and between your body's atoms that keep you from falling through the chair and, conversely, that keep the chair from passing through you.

Electromagnetic force acts through a field.

This sort of field can occur as a result of positively or negatively charged atoms (ions), atoms which have either more or fewer electrons than protons causing their overall charge to be unbalanced. Magnetic fields can also be created by applying electric current to conductive material (such as wire) with a conductive core (such as a nail).

Electric current is nothing more than a steady flow of electrons, and by turning on the current you send electrons through the core.

This aligns all the atoms in the metal so that they are parallel with each other, and this creates a magnetic field. When you turn the electric current off, the electrons stop flowing, and the atoms, no longer forced by the current to line up, cease to be magnetic.

All electromagnetic fields have a positive and a negative pole.

Even the Earth's magnetic field, which is caused by the convective forces in the planet's core, sends electrons out of its negative pole (in the geographic North Pole) and reaccepts them at its positive pole (in the geographic South Pole in Antarctica). The Earth's magnetic field, like all magnetic fields, is able to affect charged particles.

Magnetic fields move in one direction around a magnet.

This direction is always the same in relation to the flow of current from the negative to the positive poles, and it is easy to test the direction of the field using the "right hand rule." Close your fist and make a "thumbs up" sign with your right hand. The positive pole is represented by the tip of your thumb, the negative by the other end of your hand, and the direction of the magnetic field by where your closed fingers are. Thus, if you point your thumb at yourself, your magnet has current coming out its negative pole pointed towards you and looping back around to the positive pole pointed away from you, and the field is pointed counter-clockwise, which in this case is to your left.

The effects of a magnetic field do not go on forever but follow the inverse square law.

The farther you move from a magnetic field, the less its force will affect you. By moving x times away from a magnetic field, you feel $1/x2$ times less magnetism.

Closely related to the electromagnetic field is electromagnetic radiation.

This radiation can take many forms, the most familiar of which being light, radio waves that carry radio and broadcast television, microwaves that cook our food, x-rays that can image the insides or our bodies, and gamma rays that come down from space and would have killed us all long ago if it were not for the Earth's magnetic field interacting with them.

Electromagnetic radiation is created, according to James Clerk Maxwell, by the oscillations of electromagnetic fields, which create electromagnetic waves.

The wave's frequency (or how energetic it is) determines what part of the electromagnetic spectrum it occupies—whether it is a gamma ray, a blue light or a radio signal. Electromagnetic radiation is the same thing as light, with what we are used to as visible light being a range of specific frequencies within the electromagnetic spectrum, so all electromagnetic radiation moves at the speed of light.

At the quantum level, the electromagnetic force has a transfer particle moving back and forth between charged atoms, attracting and repelling them. The electromagnetic transfer particle is the photon.

Fundamental Forces: Gravity

Gravity may be the most commonly, consciously experienced force.

We can see its effects everyday when books fall off of shelves, when stray baseballs arc downwards and crash through windows and when Australians time and again fail to fall off the bottom of the world and out into space. Gravity is also largely responsible for the structure of the universe. Without it, stars would not ignite and begin fusion reactions, planets would not condense out of dust and metal and most matter would have no attraction to other matter in any way. Essentially, without gravity, life would not exist.

It may seem strange to learn that gravity is the weakest of all forces given that it holds the entire galaxy together.

Still, even with the gravitational mass of the entire planet pulling on an object such as a ball—causing it to sit motionless on the floor rather than float aimlessly off into space—a toddler could easily pick it up and run off with it, and there would be nothing the planet could do about it. Match that with the force an electromagnet exerts on metal; there is no comparison.

The idea of gravity as a force was first formulated by Isaac Newton in the late 17th century.

Newton's ideas were further elaborated on in the early 20th century by Albert Einstein, who described gravity as the effect of mass warping the fabric of space-time. This process is often portrayed as a large ball creating a divot in a flat sheet of space-time. The divot curves space-time and can catch objects that would otherwise be traveling in straight lines and redirect or even capture them.

On Earth gravity pulls objects towards the center of the planet at 9.8m/s^2.

The squared rate of time shows that gravity is by its nature a force causing acceleration. Every second, the force of gravity increases the speed of an object by an additional 9.8m/s, provided nothing able to resist the force gets in its way.

In Einstein's view of the universe, gravity moved in waves, which traveled through space at the speed of light.

As a result, he demonstrated that the force of gravity would take time to reach the object it was acting on. If, for instance, the sun were to suddenly vanish from the solar system, it would take eight minutes for the Earth to go flying off into space—the same amount of time it would take for us to stop seeing the sun's light.

Another way to view gravity is through a series of transfer particles that interact with matter and draw it closer together.

Transfer particles come into play in quantum mechanics, and they replace gravity waves as the method of spreading the force through the universe. (Actually, replace is not the right word, as quantum mechanics shows that particles and waves are really the same thing, simply looked at from different perspectives.) In quantum mechanics gravity's transfer particle is called a graviton, and it moves at the speed of light.

The farther you move from a gravitational mass, the less its force will affect you.

The drop in the gravitational force is governed by what is known as the inverse square law, which says that the attraction of any object drops in relation to the square of the distance you move from it. Essentially, if you are floating over the surface of the planet and then move x times away from it, you will feel $1/x^2$ times less gravity. So if you move 10 times farther away from where you were, you will feel 1/100 the force gravity.

Fundamental Forces: Strong and Weak Nuclear Forces

The strong and weak nuclear forces are fundamental forces, but they were discovered much later than electromagnetism and gravity primarily because they only interact with matter at a subatomic level.

Strong nuclear force is the strongest of the four fundamental forces.

Strong nuclear force is 100 times stronger than the next strongest force, electromagnetism, and 1036 times the strength of the weakest force, gravity. That said, for the thousands of years that people have been studying physics, it never occurred to anyone to even look for the strong force. That is because, despite the strong force's strength, it has such a limited range that it only interacts with matter across the distance of an atom's nucleus. In fact, its range is only about 10-15 meters, so small that the nuclei of the largest atoms—those filled with the highest number of protons and neutrons—are only just barely small enough for the strong force to keep working, making the nuclei of those atoms unstable.

The strong force was not discovered until the 1930s when scientists discovered the neutron.

Up until that time atomic nuclei were thought to consist of a collection of protons and electrons grouped together in such a way that kept them mutually attracted to each other. With the discovery of the neutron, however, a new force was needed to hold positively charged protons together with uncharged neutrons.

Strong Nuclear force interacts with Quarks.

The strong force actually does not interact directly with the protons and neutrons but with the fundamental particle that makes up protons and neutrons, quarks. Quarks come in three different color groupings: red, green and blue. (Quarks are not actually these colors; red, green and blue are just familiar names given to bits of matter that are utterly outside of our experience as humans, in order to make them easier to comprehend.) The different colors of quarks combine together to create protons and neutrons. Within each proton and neutron, the strong force holds the quarks together. That, in turn, bleeds out into the rest of the nucleus in a residual effect, holding the protons and neutrons together as well.

Like the other fundamental forces, the strong force is mediated at the quantum level using a transfer particle known as a gluon. However, unlike the transfer particles for gravity and electromagnetism (gravitons and photons, respectively), gluons have mass. It is the gluon's mass that limits the area where it can spread the strong force to only within the nucleus.

Weak nuclear force causes a type of radioactive decay.

The other fundamental force operating inside the nucleus is the weak force. The weak force causes a specific type of radioactive decay called beta decay, so named because it causes the decaying atom to emit a beta particle, which can be either an electron or a positron (a form of anti-mater also known as an anti-electron), as a by-product of changing into a different element.

Several things happen at once during beta decay, and we should look at each one individually. We saw while looking at the strong force that an atom's protons and neutrons are made up of smaller, fundamental particles called quarks, and it is the quarks that actually interact with the strong force. As it turns out, quarks are the only particle that interacts with all four fundamental forces, which means that inside the nucleus they are interacting with the weak force as well.

In addition to three different colors: red, blue and green, Quarks can be divided into six different flavors: up, down, charm, strange, top and bottom.

Before we get to how the weak force interacts with quarks, there is something else you should know about them. We mentioned above that quarks come in three different colors: red, blue and green. But they also can be divided into six different flavors: up, down, charm, strange, top and bottom. (This makes 18 different possible combinations of quark, each with a color and a flavor.) Of these flavors only up and down quarks are stable enough to form protons and neutrons.

What the weak force does is switch up quarks to down quarks and down quarks to up quarks.

This is actually the only thing the weak force does, but it has several effects. First since quarks join together to produce protons and neutrons (two up quarks and one down quark make a proton, while two down and one up quark make a neutron), the sudden change of one type of quark to another changes that combination. β– decay is beta decay where change of quarks causes a neutron to become a proton. This also causes the atom to emit an electron and a electron antineutrino. β + decay is the opposite, where a proton changes to a neutron and the atom emits a positron and an electron neutrino.

In both cases the decaying atom changes into a different kind of atom. In general, beta decay takes place in unstable isotopes (atoms that have a different number of protons and neutrons) and serves to stabilize the nucleus by equalizing the ratio of these particles. For instance, beta decay will turn the unstable plutonium 15 into far more stable strontium 16.

States of Matter

Matter on Earth can exist in three main states or phases: solid, liquid and gas. There is also a fourth phase, plasma, that occurs when matter is superheated.

The primary difference between the different phases of matter is the behavior of molecules in relation to the temperature the matter is exposed to. The lower the temperature, the closer together and more locked together the molecules are. The higher the temperature, the farther apart the molecules are and the more they move relative to one another.

Solid

Solid matter exists in a state where its molecules are locked together in a rigid

structure preventing them from moving and, as a result, solid matter is held together in a specific shape.

There are two primary types of solids, each defined by the structures in which their molecules are held. When the molecules in solid matter maintain a uniform organization they form a polycrystalline structure. This is how molecules in metal, ice and salt are organized. Polycrystalline structures are generally a result of the molecules' ionic properties. Water molecules, for instance, are formed in such a way that there are distinct ends, one with two hydrogen atoms and one with a single oxygen atom. The structure of the atoms within a water molecule means these ends are charged, giving it what amount to poles and causing water molecules to join together only in specific patterns. Under a microscope polycrystalline solids are generally described as resembling lattice work or a chain link fence, with the same pattern of molecules from one end to the other.

When molecule's electromagnetic properties do not incline them to form into particular structures, they glob together in whatever patterns they can. This produces amorphous solids, most notably foams, glass and many types of plastic. Amorphous solids have no regular pattern throughout their structure and, as a result, are poor conductors of heat and electricity.

Liquid

When solids are heated past a certain point, the electromagnetic bonds holding their molecules together loosen, and the molecules are able to move more freely.

While the temperatures required for this to happen can vary widely, the particular physical qualities of a liquid are always the same. Liquids are considered to be fluids, which differ from solids primarily in their ability to take the shape of any container they are held in. This is the result of a less intense electromagnetic connection between the molecules than there is in solids; however, there is still enough of a that liquids still want to stay all in the same place. This is why liquids still maintain a low density that is nearly identical to their densities in solid form, and why they will maintain a constant volume rather than just drift off the way gasses do.

Liquids also have a property known as viscosity, which describes their willingness to flow over and away from themselves. Liquids such as water and honey have a constant viscosity and are known as Newtonian fluids. Non-Newtonian fluids, such as a goopy mixture of water and cornstarch can change their viscosities.

Gas

The third state of matter that is commonly found on Earth is gas. Gasses are formed when matter is heated beyond its liquid state so that the electromagnetic bonds holding its molecules together are severed almost completely.

Gasses are also considered fluids and like liquids have no definite shape. But unlike liquids they also lack a definite volume and have an extremely low density compared to their solid forms.

Since gasses lack both a shape and a volume, they will expand to fill any container they are placed in. Left unbounded they will expand forever. Conversely, gasses are perfectly happy to compress together in an enclosed space. (However, the more molecules of a gas that are enclosed in a space together, the higher the gas's pressure—the force exerted by the molecules on the container's surface—will be.) One interesting thing about this expansion and compression is that it will always be homogeneous, meaning that as a gas expands to fill a container, there will never be pockets of a higher density of molecules in some areas with a lower density of molecules in others. The molecules will expand to fill the container equally.

Plasma

Plasma is the next step up from a gas; it is when a gas's molecules become super heated to the point where the molecular bonds themselves break down and the atoms begin shedding their electrons.

Although plasma is rarely found on Earth, it is the most common state of matter throughout the universe. (It is the primary state of matter in stars, for instance.) Plasma has some unique characteristics, not the least of which is that it is ionized, or electrically charged. In many ways plasma acts like a gas. It lacks any definite shape or volume, and it will homogeneously fill any container. But it is can also be manipulated by electromagnetic fields, which can be used to alter its shape or contain it. Essentially, plasma is a super-heated, magnetically charged gas.

Oxidation and Reduction

Oxidation is a chemical reaction involving the loss of electrons or the increase of the oxidation state of an element by an atom, molecule or ion.

Reduction is the opposite side of the chemical reaction that involves the gain of an electron, or the decrease in the oxidation state of an element by an ion, molecule or atom.

Originally, the word oxidation was used to refer only to the reaction of an element with oxygen to produce an oxide.

Oxygen was the first recognized oxidizing agent and thus the name oxidation. The use of the word oxidation later expanded to include reaction with any element or substances that accomplish parallel chemical reactions as that produced by oxygen. Today, oxidation is used to refer to all processes and reactions that involve a loss of electrons or an increase in the oxidation state.

The word reduction was originally used to refer to all chemical reactions that involved the loss of weight of a metallic ore or metal oxide by heating.

When a metal oxide is heated to extract the metal, oxygen is lost as a gas and the overall weight decreases. In time, it was discovered that the metallic ore or element being reduced actually gained some electrons. Today, the chemical application of the term reduction has been enlarged to include all processes and reactions that involve the gain of electrons or the decrease in the oxidation state.

Redox is a word coined from reduction and oxidation. Redox, or oxidation and reduction reactions comprise chemical reactions where the oxidation state of the atoms involved have been changed.

Redox could occur in as simple a chemical process as the oxidation process where carbon is oxidized to produce carbon dioxide (CO_2) or the use of hydrogen in the reduction of carbon to produce methane (CH_4). Redox could also occur in relatively complex reactions such as the complex process of oxidizing glucose inside the human body.

Redox reactions are primarily associated with the production of oxides with the interaction with oxygen and other such like oxidation substances. However, redox reactions would also include the transfer of electrons during the reaction process.

One peculiar characteristic of redox or oxidation and reduction reactions is that they occur as a matched set. You can thus not have an oxidation reaction, without having a corresponding reduction reaction. This is the reason why an oxidation or reduction reaction on its own is known as a half reaction. Together they both form the complete reaction because they cannot occur on their own. One side of the reaction loses electrons while the other side gains electrons during the reaction.

In is very important to note that while the loss or gain of electrons usually happens in most oxidation and reduction reactions, chemical reactions where electrons are not gained or lost can still be referred to as oxidation and reduction reactions.

The definition of oxidation and reduction reactions could thus be more accurately defined as; Oxidation is the increase in the oxidation state, and Reduction is the decrease of the oxidation state even though electrons may not always be transferred.

The transfer of electrons would usually result in the change of oxidation state, but several reactions qualify to be termed as oxidation or reduction reactions even though no electrons where transferred. A good example of these would be reactions involving chemical covalent bonds.

Speed, Acceleration and Force Problems

Acceleration

In physics, acceleration is the rate at which the velocity of a body changes with time. For example, an object such as a car that starts from a full stop, then travels in a straight line at increasing speed, is accelerating in the direction of travel. If the car changes direction at constant speed, there is strictly speaking an acceleration, although not described as such; passengers in the car will experience a force pushing them back into their seats in linear acceleration, and a sideways force on changing direction. If the speed of the car decreases, or decelerates, mathematically it is acceleration in the opposite direction. [9]

The formula for acceleration = $A = (V_f - V_0)/t$ and is measured in meters per second^2.

Here is a typical question:

A car starts from standing top and in 10 seconds is travelling 20/meters per second. What is the acceleration?

    a. 0.5 m/sec^2

    b. 1.5 m/sec^2

    c. 1 m/sec^2

    d. 2 m/sec^2

The formula for acceleration = $A = (V_f - V_0)/t$
so A = (20 m/sec - 0 m/sec)/10 sec = 2 m/sec^2

Speed

Speed is the rate of change of an objects position, or,
speed = (total distance traveled)/(total time taken).

Here is a typical question:

A rocket travels 3000 meters in 5 seconds. How fast is it travelling?

    a. 100 m/sec

    b. 200 m/sec

    c. 500 m/sec

    d. 600 m/sec

Speed = (total distance traveled)/(total time taken)
3000/5 = 600 meters per second.

Force

An everyday definition of Force is the push or pull. The more scientific definition of Force is any influence that causes an object to change its movement or direction. Force is measured in Newtons, (usually N) named after Sir Isaac Newton, and his formulation of the Second Law of motion, F = ma, where F = force, m = mass and a = acceleration.

$1 \text{ N} = 1 \text{ kg m/s}^2$.

Therefore,

Force = Mass times Acceleration Measured in Newtons.
Acceleration is the change in speed over time.
Speed is the change in position over time.

Here is a typical question:

How much force is needed to accelerate a car that weights 500 kg to 10 m/s²?

    a. 20,000 N
    b. 30,000 N
    c. 40,000 N
    d. 50,000 N

Force = Mass times Acceleration Measured in Newtons.
F = 500 X 10 = 50,000 N

Momentum

Momentum is the sum of the mass of an object and its velocity. This means that momentum measures the force produced by an object's mass and velocity.

For example, a very heavy object moving fast has a large momentum—it takes a large and prolonged force to get a very heavy object up to this speed, and it takes a large and prolonged force to bring it to a stop afterwards. If the object were lighter, or moving more slowly, then it would have less momentum, and it would be easier (i.e. require less force) to bring it to a stop.

The formula for calculating momentum is =
Momentum = mass x velocity
Or
P = MV
Where P = momentum, V = velocity and M = mass

Based on the above definition, it is clear that the momentum of a car and a bicycle both travelling at 20 m/s will not be the same, because although the velocity of the two objects are the same, their mass is different. The car would have greater momentum, due to its larger mass.

It is important to note that:

The SI unit for velocity = m/s
SI unit for Mass = kg
So therefore momentum = kg x m/s and the SI unit for momentum is kg x m/s

Momentum must always have a direction and so the final answer must reflect the direction of the momentum or velocity.

Here is a typical question:

What is the momentum of a log weighing 700 kg that is rolling down a hill at 4.6 m/s?

    a. 3220 kg x m/s down the hill

    b. 3320 kg x m/s

    c. 3320 down hill

    d. 3320 M

Answer: A

$P = MV$
$P = 700 \times 4.6$
$P = 3220$ kg x m/s down the hill.

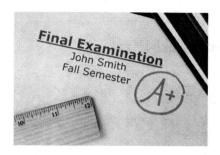

Practice Test Questions Set 1

The questions below are not exactly the same as you will find on the PAX RN - that would be too easy! And nobody knows what the questions will be and they change all the time. Below are general questions that cover the same subject areas as the PAX RN. So while the format and exact wording of the questions may differ slightly, and change from year to year, if you can answer the questions below, you will have no problem with the PAX RN.

For the best results, take this Practice Test as if it were the real exam. Set aside time when you will not be disturbed, and a location that is quiet and free of distractions. Read the instructions carefully, read each question carefully, and answer to the best of your ability.

Use the bubble answer sheets provided. When you have completed the Practice Test, check your answer against the Answer Key and read the explanation provided.

Do not attempt more than one set of practice test questions in one day. After completing the first practice test, wait two or three days before attempting the second set of questions.

Section I – Verbal Ability
Questions: 80 **Time:** 60 Minutes

Section II – Mathematics
Questions: 50 **Time:** 60 Minutes

Section III – Science
Questions: 75 **Time:** 60 minutes

Answer Sheet – Verbal Ability

1. (A) (B) (C) (D)   21. (A) (B) (C) (D)   41. (A) (B) (C) (D)   61. (A) (B) (C) (D)
2. (A) (B) (C) (D)   22. (A) (B) (C) (D)   42. (A) (B) (C) (D)   62. (A) (B) (C) (D)
3. (A) (B) (C) (D)   23. (A) (B) (C) (D)   43. (A) (B) (C) (D)   63. (A) (B) (C) (D)
4. (A) (B) (C) (D)   24. (A) (B) (C) (D)   44. (A) (B) (C) (D)   64. (A) (B) (C) (D)
5. (A) (B) (C) (D)   25. (A) (B) (C) (D)   45. (A) (B) (C) (D)   65. (A) (B) (C) (D)
6. (A) (B) (C) (D)   26. (A) (B) (C) (D)   46. (A) (B) (C) (D)   66. (A) (B) (C) (D)
7. (A) (B) (C) (D)   27. (A) (B) (C) (D)   47. (A) (B) (C) (D)   67. (A) (B) (C) (D)
8. (A) (B) (C) (D)   28. (A) (B) (C) (D)   48. (A) (B) (C) (D)   68. (A) (B) (C) (D)
9. (A) (B) (C) (D)   29. (A) (B) (C) (D)   49. (A) (B) (C) (D)   69. (A) (B) (C) (D)
10. (A) (B) (C) (D)   30. (A) (B) (C) (D)   50. (A) (B) (C) (D)   70. (A) (B) (C) (D)
11. (A) (B) (C) (D)   31. (A) (B) (C) (D)   51. (A) (B) (C) (D)   71. (A) (B) (C) (D)
12. (A) (B) (C) (D)   32. (A) (B) (C) (D)   52. (A) (B) (C) (D)   72. (A) (B) (C) (D)
13. (A) (B) (C) (D)   33. (A) (B) (C) (D)   53. (A) (B) (C) (D)   73. (A) (B) (C) (D)
14. (A) (B) (C) (D)   34. (A) (B) (C) (D)   54. (A) (B) (C) (D)   74. (A) (B) (C) (D)
15. (A) (B) (C) (D)   35. (A) (B) (C) (D)   55. (A) (B) (C) (D)   75. (A) (B) (C) (D)
16. (A) (B) (C) (D)   36. (A) (B) (C) (D)   56. (A) (B) (C) (D)   76. (A) (B) (C) (D)
17. (A) (B) (C) (D)   37. (A) (B) (C) (D)   57. (A) (B) (C) (D)   77. (A) (B) (C) (D)
18. (A) (B) (C) (D)   38. (A) (B) (C) (D)   58. (A) (B) (C) (D)   78. (A) (B) (C) (D)
19. (A) (B) (C) (D)   39. (A) (B) (C) (D)   59. (A) (B) (C) (D)   79. (A) (B) (C) (D)
20. (A) (B) (C) (D)   40. (A) (B) (C) (D)   60. (A) (B) (C) (D)   80. (A) (B) (C) (D)

Answer Sheet – Mathematics

1. Ⓐ Ⓑ Ⓒ Ⓓ
2. Ⓐ Ⓑ Ⓒ Ⓓ
3. Ⓐ Ⓑ Ⓒ Ⓓ
4. Ⓐ Ⓑ Ⓒ Ⓓ
5. Ⓐ Ⓑ Ⓒ Ⓓ
6. Ⓐ Ⓑ Ⓒ Ⓓ
7. Ⓐ Ⓑ Ⓒ Ⓓ
8. Ⓐ Ⓑ Ⓒ Ⓓ
9. Ⓐ Ⓑ Ⓒ Ⓓ
10. Ⓐ Ⓑ Ⓒ Ⓓ
11. Ⓐ Ⓑ Ⓒ Ⓓ
12. Ⓐ Ⓑ Ⓒ Ⓓ
13. Ⓐ Ⓑ Ⓒ Ⓓ
14. Ⓐ Ⓑ Ⓒ Ⓓ
15. Ⓐ Ⓑ Ⓒ Ⓓ
16. Ⓐ Ⓑ Ⓒ Ⓓ
17. Ⓐ Ⓑ Ⓒ Ⓓ

18. Ⓐ Ⓑ Ⓒ Ⓓ
19. Ⓐ Ⓑ Ⓒ Ⓓ
20. Ⓐ Ⓑ Ⓒ Ⓓ
21. Ⓐ Ⓑ Ⓒ Ⓓ
22. Ⓐ Ⓑ Ⓒ Ⓓ
23. Ⓐ Ⓑ Ⓒ Ⓓ
24. Ⓐ Ⓑ Ⓒ Ⓓ
25. Ⓐ Ⓑ Ⓒ Ⓓ
26. Ⓐ Ⓑ Ⓒ Ⓓ
27. Ⓐ Ⓑ Ⓒ Ⓓ
28. Ⓐ Ⓑ Ⓒ Ⓓ
29. Ⓐ Ⓑ Ⓒ Ⓓ
30. Ⓐ Ⓑ Ⓒ Ⓓ
31. Ⓐ Ⓑ Ⓒ Ⓓ
32. Ⓐ Ⓑ Ⓒ Ⓓ
33. Ⓐ Ⓑ Ⓒ Ⓓ
34. Ⓐ Ⓑ Ⓒ Ⓓ

35. Ⓐ Ⓑ Ⓒ Ⓓ
36. Ⓐ Ⓑ Ⓒ Ⓓ
37. Ⓐ Ⓑ Ⓒ Ⓓ
38. Ⓐ Ⓑ Ⓒ Ⓓ
39. Ⓐ Ⓑ Ⓒ Ⓓ
40. Ⓐ Ⓑ Ⓒ Ⓓ
41. Ⓐ Ⓑ Ⓒ Ⓓ
42. Ⓐ Ⓑ Ⓒ Ⓓ
43. Ⓐ Ⓑ Ⓒ Ⓓ
44. Ⓐ Ⓑ Ⓒ Ⓓ
45. Ⓐ Ⓑ Ⓒ Ⓓ
46. Ⓐ Ⓑ Ⓒ Ⓓ

Answer Sheet – Science

1. Ⓐ Ⓑ Ⓒ Ⓓ	21. Ⓐ Ⓑ Ⓒ Ⓓ	41. Ⓐ Ⓑ Ⓒ Ⓓ	61. Ⓐ Ⓑ Ⓒ Ⓓ
2. Ⓐ Ⓑ Ⓒ Ⓓ	22. Ⓐ Ⓑ Ⓒ Ⓓ	42. Ⓐ Ⓑ Ⓒ Ⓓ	62. Ⓐ Ⓑ Ⓒ Ⓓ
3. Ⓐ Ⓑ Ⓒ Ⓓ	23. Ⓐ Ⓑ Ⓒ Ⓓ	43. Ⓐ Ⓑ Ⓒ Ⓓ	63. Ⓐ Ⓑ Ⓒ Ⓓ
4. Ⓐ Ⓑ Ⓒ Ⓓ	24. Ⓐ Ⓑ Ⓒ Ⓓ	44. Ⓐ Ⓑ Ⓒ Ⓓ	64. Ⓐ Ⓑ Ⓒ Ⓓ
5. Ⓐ Ⓑ Ⓒ Ⓓ	25. Ⓐ Ⓑ Ⓒ Ⓓ	45. Ⓐ Ⓑ Ⓒ Ⓓ	65. Ⓐ Ⓑ Ⓒ Ⓓ
6. Ⓐ Ⓑ Ⓒ Ⓓ	26. Ⓐ Ⓑ Ⓒ Ⓓ	46. Ⓐ Ⓑ Ⓒ Ⓓ	66. Ⓐ Ⓑ Ⓒ Ⓓ
7. Ⓐ Ⓑ Ⓒ Ⓓ	27. Ⓐ Ⓑ Ⓒ Ⓓ	47. Ⓐ Ⓑ Ⓒ Ⓓ	67. Ⓐ Ⓑ Ⓒ Ⓓ
8. Ⓐ Ⓑ Ⓒ Ⓓ	28. Ⓐ Ⓑ Ⓒ Ⓓ	48. Ⓐ Ⓑ Ⓒ Ⓓ	68. Ⓐ Ⓑ Ⓒ Ⓓ
9. Ⓐ Ⓑ Ⓒ Ⓓ	29. Ⓐ Ⓑ Ⓒ Ⓓ	49. Ⓐ Ⓑ Ⓒ Ⓓ	69. Ⓐ Ⓑ Ⓒ Ⓓ
10. Ⓐ Ⓑ Ⓒ Ⓓ	30. Ⓐ Ⓑ Ⓒ Ⓓ	50. Ⓐ Ⓑ Ⓒ Ⓓ	70. Ⓐ Ⓑ Ⓒ Ⓓ
11. Ⓐ Ⓑ Ⓒ Ⓓ	31. Ⓐ Ⓑ Ⓒ Ⓓ	51. Ⓐ Ⓑ Ⓒ Ⓓ	71. Ⓐ Ⓑ Ⓒ Ⓓ
12. Ⓐ Ⓑ Ⓒ Ⓓ	32. Ⓐ Ⓑ Ⓒ Ⓓ	52. Ⓐ Ⓑ Ⓒ Ⓓ	72. Ⓐ Ⓑ Ⓒ Ⓓ
13. Ⓐ Ⓑ Ⓒ Ⓓ	33. Ⓐ Ⓑ Ⓒ Ⓓ	53. Ⓐ Ⓑ Ⓒ Ⓓ	73. Ⓐ Ⓑ Ⓒ Ⓓ
14. Ⓐ Ⓑ Ⓒ Ⓓ	34. Ⓐ Ⓑ Ⓒ Ⓓ	54. Ⓐ Ⓑ Ⓒ Ⓓ	74. Ⓐ Ⓑ Ⓒ Ⓓ
15. Ⓐ Ⓑ Ⓒ Ⓓ	35. Ⓐ Ⓑ Ⓒ Ⓓ	55. Ⓐ Ⓑ Ⓒ Ⓓ	75. Ⓐ Ⓑ Ⓒ Ⓓ
16. Ⓐ Ⓑ Ⓒ Ⓓ	36. Ⓐ Ⓑ Ⓒ Ⓓ	56. Ⓐ Ⓑ Ⓒ Ⓓ	76. Ⓐ Ⓑ Ⓒ Ⓓ
17. Ⓐ Ⓑ Ⓒ Ⓓ	37. Ⓐ Ⓑ Ⓒ Ⓓ	57. Ⓐ Ⓑ Ⓒ Ⓓ	77. Ⓐ Ⓑ Ⓒ Ⓓ
18. Ⓐ Ⓑ Ⓒ Ⓓ	38. Ⓐ Ⓑ Ⓒ Ⓓ	58. Ⓐ Ⓑ Ⓒ Ⓓ	78. Ⓐ Ⓑ Ⓒ Ⓓ
19. Ⓐ Ⓑ Ⓒ Ⓓ	39. Ⓐ Ⓑ Ⓒ Ⓓ	59. Ⓐ Ⓑ Ⓒ Ⓓ	79. Ⓐ Ⓑ Ⓒ Ⓓ
20. Ⓐ Ⓑ Ⓒ Ⓓ	40. Ⓐ Ⓑ Ⓒ Ⓓ	60. Ⓐ Ⓑ Ⓒ Ⓓ	80. Ⓐ Ⓑ Ⓒ Ⓓ

Section I - Verbal Ability

Directions: The following questions are based on a number of reading passages. Each passage is followed by a series of questions. Read each passage carefully, and then answer the questions based on it. You may reread the passage as often as you wish. When you have finished answering the questions based on one passage, go right on to the next passage. Choose the best answer based on the information given and implied.

Questions 1 – 4 refer to the following passage.

Passage 1 - Infectious Disease

An infectious disease is a clinically evident illness resulting from the presence of pathogenic agents, such as viruses, bacteria, fungi, protozoa, multi cellular parasites, and unusual proteins known as prions. Infectious pathologies are also called communicable diseases or transmissible diseases, due to their potential of transmission from one person or species to another by a replicating agent (as opposed to a toxin).

Transmission of an infectious disease can occur in many different ways. Physical contact, liquids, food, body fluids, contaminated objects, and airborne inhalation can all transmit infecting agents.

Transmissible diseases that occur through contact with an ill person, or objects touched by them, are especially infective, and are sometimes referred to as contagious diseases. Communicable diseases that require a more specialized route of infection, such as through blood or needle transmission, or sexual transmission, are usually not regarded as contagious.

The term infectivity describes the ability of an organism to enter, survive and multiply in the host, while the infectiousness of a disease indicates the comparative ease with which the disease is transmitted. An infection however, is not synonymous with an infectious disease, as an infection may not cause important clinical symptoms. [10]

1. What can we infer from the first paragraph in this passage?

    a. Sickness from a toxin can be easily transmitted from one person to another.

    b. Sickness from an infectious disease can be easily transmitted from one person to another.

    c. Few sicknesses are transmitted from one person to another.

    d. Infectious diseases are easily treated.

2. What are two other names for infections' pathologies?

    a. Communicable diseases or transmissible diseases

    b. Communicable diseases or terminal diseases

    c. Transmissible diseases or preventable diseases

    d. Communicative diseases or unstable diseases

3. What does infectivity describe?

    a. The inability of an organism to multiply in the host.

    b. The inability of an organism to reproduce.

    c. The ability of an organism to enter, survive and multiply in the host.

    d. The ability of an organism to reproduce in the host.

4. How do we know an infection is not synonymous with an infectious disease?

    a. Because an infectious disease destroys infections with enough time.

    b. Because an infection may not cause important clinical symptoms or impair host function.

    c. We do not. The two are synonymous.

    d. Because an infection is too fatal to be an infectious disease.

Questions 5 – 8 refer to the following passage.

Passage 2 - Viruses

A virus (from the Latin virus meaning toxin or poison) is a small infectious agent that can replicate only inside the living cells of other organisms. Most viruses are too small to be seen directly with a microscope. Viruses infect all types of organisms, from animals and plants to bacteria and single-celled organisms.

Unlike prions and viroids, viruses consist of two or three parts: all viruses have genes made from either DNA or RNA, all have a protein coat that protects these genes, and some have an envelope of fat that surrounds them when they are outside a cell. (Viroids do not have a protein coat and prions contain no RNA or DNA.) Viruses vary from simple to very complex structures. Most viruses are about one hundred times smaller than an average bacterium. The origins of viruses in the evolutionary history of life are unclear: some may have evolved from plasmids—pieces of DNA that can move between cells—while others may have evolved from bacteria.

Viruses spread in many ways; plant viruses are often transmitted from plant to plant by insects that feed on sap, such as aphids, while animal viruses can be carried by blood-sucking insects. These disease-bearing organisms are known as vectors. Influenza viruses are spread by coughing and sneezing. HIV is one of several viruses transmitted through sexual contact and by exposure to infected blood. Viruses can infect only a limited range of host cells called the "host range". This can be broad as when a virus is capable of infecting many species or narrow. [11]

5. What can we infer from the first paragraph in this selection?

     a. A virus is the same as bacterium

     b. A person with excellent vision can see a virus with the naked eye

     c. A virus cannot be seen with the naked eye

     d. Not all viruses are dangerous

6. What types of organisms do viruses infect?

     a. Only plants and humans

     b. Only animals and humans

     c. Only disease-prone humans

     d. All types of organisms

7. How many parts do prions and viroids consist of?

     a. Two

     b. Three

     c. Either less than two or more than three

     d. Less than two

8. What is one common virus spread by coughing and sneezing?

     a. AIDS

     b. Influenza

     c. Herpes

     d. Tuberculosis

Questions 9 – 11 refer to the following passage.

Passage 3 – Clouds

The first stage of a thunderstorm is the cumulus stage, or developing stage. In this stage, masses of moisture are lifted upwards into the atmosphere. The trigger for this lift can be insulation heating the ground producing thermals, areas where two winds converge, forcing air upwards, or where winds blow over terrain of increasing elevation. Moisture in the air rapidly cools into liquid drops of water, which appears as cumulus clouds.

As the water vapor condenses into liquid, latent heat is released which warms the air, causing it to become less dense than the surrounding dry air. The warm air rises in an updraft through the process of convection (hence the term convective precipitation). This creates a low-pressure zone beneath the forming thunderstorm. In a typical thunderstorm, approximately 5×10^8 kg of water vapor is lifted, and the amount of energy released when this condenses is about equal to the energy used by a city of 100,000 in a month. [12]

9. The cumulus stage of a thunderstorm is the

   a. The last stage of the storm.
   b. The middle stage of the storm formation.
   c. The beginning of the thunderstorm.
   d. The period after the thunderstorm has ended.

10. One of the ways the air is warmed is

   a. Air moving downwards, which creates a high-pressure zone.
   b. Air cooling and becoming less dense, causing it to rise.
   c. Moisture moving downward toward the earth.
   d. Heat created by water vapor condensing into liquid.

11. Identify the correct sequence of events.

   a. Warm air rises, water droplets condense, creating more heat, and the air rises further.
   b. Warm air rises and cools, water droplets condense, causing low pressure.
   c. Warm air rises and collects water vapor, the water vapor condenses as the air rises, which creates heat, and causes the air to rise further.
   d. None of the above.

Questions 12 – 14 refer to the following passage.

Passage 4 – US Weather Service

The United States National Weather Service classifies thunderstorms as severe when they reach a predetermined level. Usually, this means the storm is strong enough to inflict wind or hail damage. In most of the United States, a storm is considered severe if winds reach over 50 knots (58 mph or 93 km/h), hail is ¾ inch (2 cm) diameter or larger, or if meteorologists report funnel clouds or tornadoes. In the Central Region of the

United States National Weather Service, the hail threshold for a severe thunderstorm is 1 inch (2.5 cm) in diameter. Though a funnel cloud or tornado indicates the presence of a severe thunderstorm, the various meteorological agencies would issue a tornado warning rather than a severe thunderstorm warning in this case.

Meteorologists in Canada define a severe thunderstorm as either having tornadoes, wind gusts of 90 km/h or greater, hail 2 centimeters in diameter or greater, rainfall more than 50 millimeters in 1 hour, or 75 millimeters in 3 hours.

Severe thunderstorms can develop from any type of thunderstorm. [14]

12. What is the purpose of this passage?

    a. Explaining when a thunderstorm turns into a tornado

    b. Explaining who issues storm warnings, and when these warnings should be issued

    c. Explaining when meteorologists consider a thunderstorm severe

    d. None of the above

13. It is possible to infer from this passage that

    a. Different areas and countries have different criteria for determining a severe storm.

    b. Thunderstorms can include lightning and tornadoes, as well as violent winds and large hail.

    c. If someone spots both a thunderstorm and a tornado, meteorological agencies will immediately issue a severe storm warning.

    d. Canada has a much different alert system for severe storms, with criteria that are far less.

14. What would the Central Region of the United States National Weather Service do if hail was 2.7 cm in diameter?

    a. Not issue a severe thunderstorm warning.

    b. Issue a tornado warning.

    c. Issue a severe thunderstorm warning.

    d. Sleet must also accompany the hail before the Weather Service will issue a storm warning.

Questions 15 – 18 refer to the following passage.

Passage 5 – Clouds

A cloud is a visible mass of droplets or frozen crystals floating in the atmosphere above the surface of the Earth or other planetary bodies. Another type of cloud is a mass of material in space, attracted by gravity, called interstellar clouds and nebulae. The branch of meteorology which studies clouds is called nephrology. When we are speaking of Earth clouds, water vapor is usually the condensing substance, which forms small droplets or ice crystal. These crystals are typically 0.01 mm in diameter. Dense, deep clouds reflect most light, so they appear white, at least from the top. Cloud droplets scatter light very efficiently, so the further into a cloud light travels, the weaker it gets. This accounts for the gray or dark appearance at the base of large clouds. Thin clouds may appear to have acquired the color of their environment or background. [12]

15. What are clouds made of?

    a. Water droplets

    b. Ice crystals

    c. Ice crystals and water droplets

    d. Clouds on Earth are made of ice crystals and water droplets

16. The main idea of this passage is

    a. Condensation occurs in clouds, having an intense effect on the weather on the surface of the earth.

    b. Atmospheric gases are responsible for the gray color of clouds just before a severe storm happens.

    c. A cloud is a visible mass of droplets or frozen crystals floating in the atmosphere above the surface of the Earth or other planetary body.

    d. Clouds reflect light in varying amounts and degrees, depending on the size and concentration of the water droplets.

17. The branch of meteorology that studies clouds is called

    a. Convection

    b. Thermal meteorology

    c. Nephology

    d. Nephelometry

18. Why are clouds white on top and grey on the bottom?

a. Because water droplets inside the cloud do not reflect light, it appears white, and the further into the cloud the light travels, the less light is reflected making the bottom appear dark.

b. Because water droplets outside the cloud reflect light, it appears dark, and the further into the cloud the light travels, the more light is reflected making the bottom appear white.

c. Because water droplets inside the cloud reflects light, making it appear white, and the further into the cloud the light travels, the more light is reflected making the bottom appear dark.

d. None of the above.

Questions 19 - 22 refer to the following recipe.

Chocolate Chip Cookies

3/4 cup sugar
3/4 cup packed brown sugar
1 cup butter, softened
2 large eggs, beaten
1 teaspoon vanilla extract
2 1/4 cups all-purpose flour
1 teaspoon baking soda
3/4 teaspoon salt
2 cups semisweet chocolate chips

If desired, 1 cup chopped pecans, or chopped walnuts.
Preheat oven to 375 degrees.

Mix sugar, brown sugar, butter, vanilla and eggs in a large bowl. Stir in flour, baking soda, and salt. The dough will be very stiff.

Stir in chocolate chips by hand with a sturdy wooden spoon. Add the pecans, or other nuts, if desired. Stir until the chocolate chips and nuts are evenly dispersed.

Drop dough by rounded tablespoonfuls 2 inches apart onto a cookie sheet.

Bake 8 to 10 minutes or until light brown. Cookies may look underdone, but they will finish cooking after you take them out of the oven.

19. What is the correct order for adding these ingredients?

    a. Brown sugar, baking soda, chocolate chips

    b. Baking soda, brown sugar, chocolate chips

    c. Chocolate chips, baking soda, brown sugar

    d. Baking soda, chocolate chips, brown sugar

20. What does sturdy mean?

    a. Long

    b. Strong

    c. Short

    d. Wide

21. What does disperse mean?

    a. Scatter

    b. To form a ball

    c. To stir

    d. To beat

22. When can you stop stirring the nuts?

    a. When the cookies are cooked

    b. When the nuts are evenly distributed

    c. As soon as the nuts are added

    d. After the chocolate chips are added

Questions 23 – 25 refer to the following passage.

Passage 7 – Caterpillars

Butterfly larvae, or caterpillars, eat enormous quantities of leaves and spend practically all their time in search of food. Although most caterpillars are herbivorous, a few species eat other insects. Some larvae form mutual associations with ants. They communicate with ants using vibrations transmitted through the soil, as well as with chemical signals. The ants provide some degree of protection to the larvae and they in turn gather honeydew secretions. [13]

23. What do most larvae spend their time looking for?

    a. Leaves

    b. Insects

    c. Leaves and insects

    d. Honeydew secretions

24. What benefit do larvae get from association with ants?

    a. They do not receive any benefit

    b. Ants give them protection

    c. Ants give them food

    d. Ants give them honeydew secretions

25. Do ants or larvae benefit most from association?

    a. Ants benefit most

    b. Larvae benefit most

    c. Both benefit the same

    d. Neither benefits

Questions 26 – 30 refer to the following passage.

Passage 8 – Navy Seals

The United States Navy's Sea, Air and Land Teams, commonly known as Navy SEALs, are the U.S. Navy's principal special operations force, and a part of the Naval Special Warfare Command (NSWC) as well as the maritime component of the United States Special Operations Command (USSOCOM).

The unit's acronym ("SEAL") comes from their capacity to operate at sea, in the air, and on land – but it is their ability to work underwater that separates SEALs from most other military units in the world. Navy SEALs are trained and have been deployed in a wide variety of missions, including direct action and special reconnaissance operations, unconventional warfare, foreign internal defence, hostage rescue, counter-terrorism and other missions. All SEALs are members of either the United States Navy or the United States Coast Guard.

In the early morning of May 2, 2011 local time, a team of 40 CIA-led Navy SEALs completed an operation to kill Osama bin Laden in Abbottabad, Pakistan about 35 miles (56 km) from Islamabad, the country's capital. The Navy SEALs were part of the Naval Special Warfare Development Group, previously called "Team 6". President Barack Obama later confirmed the death of bin Laden. The unprecedented media coverage raised the public profile of the SEAL community, particularly the counter-terrorism specialists commonly known as SEAL Team 6. [14]

26. Are Navy SEALs part of USSOCOM?

a. Yes

b. No

c. Only for special operations

d. No, they are part of the US Navy

27. What separates Navy SEALs from other military units?

a. Belonging to NSWC

b. Direct action and special reconnaissance operations

c. Working underwater

d. Working for other military units in the world

28. What other military organizations do SEALs belong to?

a. The US Navy

b. The Coast Guard

c. The US Army

d. The Navy and the Coast Guard

29. What other organization participated in the Bin Laden raid?

a. The CIA

b. The US Military

c. Counter-terrorism specialists

d. None of the above

30. What is the new name for Team 6?

a. They were always called Team 6

b. The counter-terrorism specialists

c. The Naval Special Warfare Development Group

d. None of the above

Questions 31 – 34 refer to the following passage.

Passage 9 - Gardening

Gardening for food extends far into prehistory. Ornamental gardens were known in ancient times, a famous example being the Hanging Gardens of Babylon, while ancient Rome had dozens of gardens.

The earliest forms of gardens emerged from the people's need to grow herbs and vegetables. It was only later that rich individuals created gardens for purely decorative purposes.

In ancient Egypt, rich people created ornamental gardens to relax in the shade of the trees. Egyptians believed that gods liked gardens. Commonly, walls surrounded ancient Egyptian gardens with trees planted in rows.

The most popular tree species were date palms, sycamores, fig trees, nut trees, and willows. In addition to ornamental gardens, wealthy Egyptians kept vineyards to produce wine.

The Assyrians are also known for their beautiful gardens in what we know today as Iraq. Assyrian gardens were very large, with some of them used for hunting and others as leisure gardens. Cypress and palm were the most popular trees in Assyrian gardens.[38]

31. Why did wealthy people in Egypt have gardens?

    a. For food

    b. To relax in the shade

    c. For ornamentation

    d. For hunting

32. What did the Egyptians believe about gardens?

    a. They believed gods loved gardens.

    b. They believed gods hated gardens.

    c. The didn't have any beliefs about gods and gardens.

    d. They believed gods hated trees.

33. What kinds of trees did the Assyrians like?

a. The Assyrians liked date palms, sycamores, fig trees, nut trees, and willows.

b. The Assyrians liked Cypresses and palms.

c. The Assyrians didn't like trees.

d. The Assyrians liked hedges and vines.

34. Which came first, gardening for vegetables or ornamental gardens?

a. Ornamental gardens came before vegetable gardens.

b. Vegetable gardens came before ornamental gardens.

c. Vegetable and ornamental gardens appeared at the same time.

d. The passage does not give enough information.

Questions 35 – 38 refer to the following passage.

Passage 10 - Gardens

Ancient Roman gardens are known for their statues and sculptures, which were never missing from the lives of Romans. Romans designed their gardens with hedges and vines as well as a wide variety of flowers, including acanthus, cornflowers and crocus, cyclamen, hyacinth, iris and ivy, lavender, lilies, myrtle, narcissus, poppy, rosemary and violet. Flower beds were popular in the courtyards of the rich Romans.

The Middle Ages was a period of decline in gardening. After the fall of Rome, gardening was only for the purpose of growing medicinal herbs and decorating church altars.

Islamic gardens were built after the model of Persian gardens, with enclosed walls and watercourses dividing the garden into four. Commonly, the center of the garden would have a pool or pavilion. Mosaics and glazed tiles used to decorate elaborate fountains are specific to Islamic gardens. [15]

35. What is a characteristic feature of Roman gardens?

a. Statues and sculptures

b. Flower beds

c. Medicinal herbs

d. Courtyard gardens

36. When did gardening decline?

a. Before the Fall of Rome

b. Gardening did not decline

c. Before the Middle Ages

d. After the Fall of Rome

37. What kind of gardening was done during the Middle Ages?

a. Gardening with hedges and vines

b. Gardening with a wide variety of flowers

c. Gardening for herbs and church alters

d. Gardening divided by watercourses

38. What is a characteristic feature of Islamic Gardens?

a. Statues and Sculptures

b. Decorative tiles and fountains

c. Herbs

d. Flower beds

Questions 39 – 42 refer to the following passage.

Passage 11 - Coral Reefs

Coral reefs are underwater structures made from calcium carbonate secreted by corals. Corals are colonies of tiny animals found in marine waters that contain few nutrients. Most coral reefs are built from a type of coral called stony corals or Scleractinia, which in turn consist of polyps that cluster in groups. The polyps are like tiny sea anemones, which they are closely related. But unlike sea anemones, coral polyps secrete hard carbonate exoskeletons which support and protect their bodies. Reefs grow best in warm, shallow, clear, sunny and agitated waters. They are most commonly found in shallow tropical waters, but deep water and cold water corals also exist on smaller scales in other areas.

Often called "rainforests of the sea", coral reefs form some of the most diverse ecosystems on Earth. They occupy less than one tenth of one percent of the world's ocean surface, about half the area of France, yet they provide a home for twenty-five percent of all marine species.

Paradoxically, coral reefs flourish even though they are surrounded by ocean waters that provide few nutrients. [39]

39. Why are coral reefs called rainforests of the sea?

a. Because they are so colorful

b. Because they are a diverse ecosystem

c. Because they look like rainforests

d. Because occupy less than one tenth of one percent of the world's ocean surface

40. What marine animal are corals closely related to?

a. Sea Anemones

b. Polyps

c. Sea Polyps

d. Anemones and Polyps

41. Where are coral reefs found?

a. In freshwater with few nutrients

b. In marine water with a lot of nutrients

c. In marine waters with few nutrients

d. In marine water with no nutrients

42. Where do corals reefs grow?

a. Hot deep water

b. Clear, warm still water

c. Warm agitated water

d. Warm, clear, shallow and agitated water

Verbal Ability Part II – Vocabulary

43. Choose a verb that means fearless or invulnerable to intimidation and fear.

a. Feeble

b. Strongest

c. Dauntless

d. Super

44. Choose a word that means the same as the underlined word.

I see the differences when they are placed side-by-side and <u>juxtaposed.</u>

a. Compared

b. Eliminated

c. Overturned

d. Exonerated

45. Choose the best definition of regicide.

a. v. To endow or furnish with requisite ability, character, knowledge and skill

b. n. killing of a king

c. adj. Disposed to seize by violence or by unlawful or greedy methods

d. v. To refresh after labor

46. Choose the best definition of pernicious.

a. Deadly

b. Infectious

c. Common

d. Rare

47. Fill in the blank.

After she received her influenza vaccination, Nan thought that she was _____ to the common cold.

    a. Immune

    b. Susceptible

    c. Vulnerable

    d. At risk

48. Choose a word that means the same as the underlined word.

She performed the gymnastics and stretches so well! I have never seen anyone so <u>nimble</u>.

    a. Awkward

    b. Agile

    c. Quick

    d. Taut

49. Choose a word that means the same as the underlined word.

Are there any more <u>queries</u>? We have already had so many questions today.

    a. Questions

    b. Commands

    c. Obfuscations

    d. Paradoxes

50. Choose a verb that means to remove a leader or high official from position.

    a. Sack

    b. Suspend

    c. Depose

    d. Dropped

51. Choose the best definition of pedestrian.

    a. Rare

    b. Often

    c. Walking or Running

    d. Commonplace

52. Choose the best definition of petulant.

    a. Patient

    b. Childish

    c. Impatient

    d. Mature

53. Fill in the blank.

Paul's rose bushes were being destroyed by Japanese beetles, so he invested in a good _____.

    a. Fungicide

    b. Fertilizer

    c. Sprinkler

    d. Pesticide

54. Choose the best definition of salient.

    a. v. To make light by fermentation, as dough

    b. adj. Not stringent or energetic

    c. adj. negligible

    d. adj. worthy of note or relevant

55. Choose the best definition of sedentary.

    a. n. A morbid condition, due to obstructed excretion of bile or characterized by yellowing of the skin

    b. adj. not moving or sitting at a place

    c. v. To wander from place to place

    d. n. Perplexity

56. Fill in the blank.

The last time that the crops failed, the entire nation experienced months of _____.

    a. Famine

    b. Harvest

    c. Plenitude

    d. Disease

57. Choose the best definition of stint.

    a. Thrifty

    b. Annoyed

    c. Dislike

    d. Insult

58. Choose the best definition of precipitate.

    a. To rain

    b. To throw down

    c. To throw up

    d. to snow

59. Choose the verb that means to build up or strengthen in relation to morals or religion.

    a. Sanctify

    b. Amplify

    c. Edify

    d. Wry

60. Choose the noun that means exit or way out.

    a. Door-jamb

    b. Egress

    c. Regress

    d. Furtherance

61. Choose the best definition of the underlined word.

The tide was in this morning but now it is starting to <u>recede</u>.

    a. Go out

    b. Flow

    c. Swell

    d. Come in

62. Choose the word that means private, personal.

    a. Confidential

    b. Hysteric

    c. Simplistic

    d. Promissory

63. Choose the best definition of the underlined word.

I don't think that will make it any better - it is just going to <u>aggravate</u> the situation.

    a. Worsen

    b. Precipitate

    c. Elongate

    d. None of the above

64. Choose the best definition of the underlined word.

I didn't think this was her first appearance, but it is her <u>debut</u>.

    a. Exit

    b. Introduction

    c. Curtain Call

    d. Resignation

65. Fill in the blank.

Because of a pituitary dysfunction, Karl lacked the necessary _____ to grow as tall as his father.

    a. Glands

    b. Hormones

    c. Vitamins

    d. Testosterone

66. Choose the best definition of importune.

    a. To find an opportunity

    b. To ask all the time

    c. Cannot find an opportunity

    d. None of the above

67. Choose the best definition of sedulous.

    a. n. The support on or against which a lever rests

    b. adj. constant steady pursuit

    c. v. To oppose with an equal force

    d. n. The branch of medical science that relates to improving health

68. Choose the best definition of tincture.

    a. n. alcoholic drink with plant extract used for medicine

    b. n. An artificial trance-sleep

    c. n. a special medicinal drink made by mixing water with plant extracts

    d. adj. the point of puncture

69. Choose the noun that means serious criminal offence that is punishable by death or imprisonment above a year

    a. Trespass

    b. Hampers

    c. Felony

    d. Obligatory

70. Choose the best meaning of the underlined word.

His library is enormous. I didn't realize he was such a <u>bibliophile</u>.

    a. Book lover

    b. Audiophile

    c. Bibliophobe

    d. Audiophobe

71. Fill in the blank.

When Mr. Davis returned from southern Asia, he told us about the _____ that sometimes swept the area, bringing torrential rain.

    a. Monsoons

    b. Hurricanes

    c. Blizzards

    d. Floods

72. Choose the best definition of volatile.

    a. Not explosive

    b. Catches fire easily

    c. Does not catch fire

    d. Explosive

73. Choose the word that means the same as plaintive.

    a. Happy

    b. Mournful

    c. Faint

    d. Plain

74. What is the best definition of truism?

    a. n. A comparison which directs the mind to the representative object itself

    b. n. self evident or clear obvious truth

    c. n. a statement that is true but that can hardly be proved

    d. n. false statements

75. Choose the verb that means to encourage or incite troublesome acts.

    a. Comment

    b. Foment

    c. Integument

    d. Atonement

76. Choose the adjective that means dignified, solemn that is appropriate for a funeral.

    a. Funereal

    b. Prediction

    c. Wailing

    d. Vociferous

77. Choose the best definition for the underlined word.

I thought they were being very discreet, but they were, in fact, very <u>flagrant</u>.

    a. Obvious

    b. Secretive

    c. Hidden

    d. Subtle

78. Fill in the blank.

Is it true that _____ always grows on the north side of trees?

    a. Lichens

    b. Moss

    c. Ferns

    d. Ground cover

79. Choose the best definition of nexus.

    a. A connection

    b. A telephone switch

    c. Part of a computer

    d. None of the above.

80. Choose the best definition of zealot.

    a. n. a person who is very passionate and fanatic about his specific objectives or beliefs

    b. n. The property or state of allowing the passage of light

    c. adj. Existing for a short time only

    d. n. An interpreter

Section II – Math

1. What is 1/3 of 3/4?

    a. 1/4

    b. 1/3

    c. 2/3

    d. 3/4

2. What fraction of $1500 is $75?

    a. 1/14

    b. 3/5

    c. 7/10

    d. 1/20

3. Add $-3x^2 + 2x + 6$ and $-x^2 - x - 1$.

    a. $-2x^2 + x + 5$

    b. $-4x^2 + x + 5$

    c. $-2x^2 + 3x + 5$

    d. $-4x^2 + 3x + 5$

4. 3.14 + 2.73 + 23.7 =

    a. 28.57

    b. 30.57

    c. 29.56

    d. 29.57

5. Find the mean of these set of numbers – 200,000, 10,020, 30,000, 15,000 1080

    a. 1080

    b. 15,000

    c. 256,100

    d. 51,220

6. What is 0.27 + 0.33 expressed as a fraction?

    a. 3/6

    b. 4/7

    c. 3/5

    d. 2/7

7. What is (3.13 + 7.87) X 5?

    a. 65

    b. 50

    c. 45

    d. 55

8. Express 3^4 in standard form

    a. 81

    b. 27

    c. 12

    d. 9

9. What is 2/4 X 3/4 reduced to lowest terms?

    a. 6/12

    b. 3/8

    c. 6/16

    d. 3/4

10. If a = 2 and y = 5, solve $xy^3 - x^3$

    a. 240

    b. 258

    c. 248

    d. 242

11. Three tenths of 90 equals:

    a. 18

    b. 45

    c. 27

    d. 36

12. Find the mean of these set of numbers – 1, 2, 3, 4, 5, 6, 7, 8, 9, 10

    a. 55

    b. 5.5

    c. 11

    d. 10

13. .4% of 36 equals

    a. 1.44

    b. .144

    c. 14.4

    d. 144

14. 5x + 3 = 7x -1. Find x

    a. 1/3

    b. 1/2

    c. 1

    d. 2

15. Find 2 numbers that sum to 21 and the sum of the squares is 261.

    a. 14 and 7

    b. 15 and 6

    c. 16 and 5

    d. 17 and 4

16. 5x + 2(x + 7) = 14x – 7. Find x

    a. 1

    b. 2

    c. 3

    d. 4

17. 5(z + 1) = 3(z + 2) + 11. Find z

    a. 2

    b. 4

    c. 6

    d. 12

18. What are the prime factors of 81?

    a. 3 x 3 x 9

    b. 3 x 27

    c. 3 x 3 x 3 x 3

    d. All of the above

19. The price of a book went up from $20 to $25. What percent did the price increase?

    a. 5%

    b. 10%

    c. 20%

    d. 25%

20. After taking several practice tests, Brian improved the results of his GRE test by 30%. Given that the first time he took the test Brian answered 150 questions correctly, how many questions did he answer correctly on the second test?

    a. 105

    b. 120

    c. 180

    d. 195

21. Simplify $4^3 + 2^4$

    a. 45

    b. 108

    c. 80

    d. 48

22. A square lawn has an area of 62,500 square meters. How much will it cost to build a fence around it at a rate of $5.5 per meter?

    a. $4000

    b. $4500

    c. $5000

    d. $5500

23. A javelin is thrown into a field at 18m/s. if the Javelin weighs 1.5kg, what is the momentum?

    a. 1.2 kg x m/s into the field

    b. 12 kg x m/s into the field

    c. 27 kg x m/s into the field

    d. 2.7 kg x m/s into the field

24. Convert 204 to scientific notation

    a. 2.04×10^{-2}

    b. 0.204×10^2

    c. 2.04×10^3

    d. 2.04×10^2

25. There are 15 yellow and 35 orange balls in a basket. How many yellow balls must be added to make the yellow balls 65%?

    a. 35

    b. 50

    c. 65

    d. 70

26. If 144 students need to go on a trip and the buses each carry 36 students, how many buses are needed?

    a. 2

    b. 3

    c. 4

    d. 4.5

27. Using the factoring method, solve the quadratic equation: $x^2 + 4x + 4 = 0$

      a. 0 and 1

      b. 1 and 2

      c. 2

      d. -2

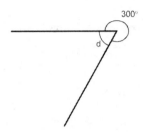

28. What is the measurement of the indicated angle?

      a. 45°

      b. 90°

      c. 60°

      d. 50°

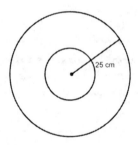

29. What is the distance travelled by the wheel above, when it makes 175 revolutions?

      a. 87.5 π m

      b. 875 π m

      c. 8.75 π m

      d. 8750 π m

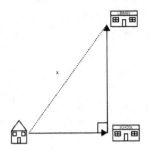

30. Every day starting from his home Peter travels due east to the school. After school he travels due north to the library. This way Peter travels 25 kilometers. What is the distance between Peter's home and the library?

      a. 15 km

      b. 10 km

      c. 5 km

      d. 12 ½ km

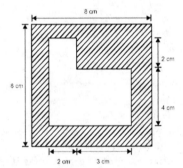

31. What is the area of the shaded region in the figure above?

      a. 64 cm²

      b. 44 cm²

      c. 60 cm²

      d. 40 cm²

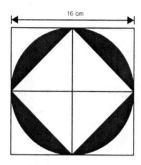

32. A tile factory makes custom tiles, shown above, from two types of stone. If a customer requires 200 tiles, how much black stone will be required?

    a. 256 m²

    b. 2560 m²

    c. 2.56 m²

    d. 25.6 m²

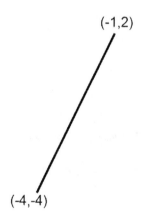

33. What is the slope of the line above?

    a. 1

    b. 2

    c. 3

    d. -2

34. A caterer is hired for a wedding and needs to calculate how much wine is needed. The couple for her weddings always gets two liters of wine. Each guest receives 0.20 liters. If y is the amount of wine needed in total liters, and if x is the number of wedding guests, which equation below should be used to figure out the number of liters the caterer will need?

    a. y = 0.20x + 2

    b. y = 2x + 0.20

    c. y = 2.20x

    d. x = 0.20y + 2

35. If we know it takes 12 men to operate four machines, how many are required for 20 machines?

    a. 6

    b. 20

    c. 60

    d. 9

36. Brad has agreed to buy everyone a Coke. Each drink costs $1.89, and there are 5 friends. Estimate Brad's cost.

    a. $7

    b. $8

    c. $10

    d. $12

37. An object that weighs 500g is rolling along the road at 3.5m/s, what is the momentum of the object?

    a. 124.9 kg x m/s along road

    b. 17. 50 kg x m/s along road

    c. 1750 kg x m/s along road

    d. 1.75 kg x m/s along road

38. Solve √121

    A. 11
    B. 12
    C. 21
    D. None of the above

39. What are the prime factors of 25?

    a. 4 x 5.5
    b. 5 x 5 x 5
    c. 1 x 25
    d. 5 x 5

40. Convert 0.00002011 to scientific notation

    a. 2.011×10^{-4}
    b. 2.011×10^{5}
    c. 2.011×10^{-6}
    d. 2.011×10^{-5}

41. Express the ratio of 7:25 as a percentage.

    a. 20%
    b. 22%
    c. 25%
    d. 28%

42.

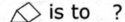

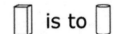

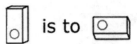

43.

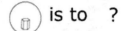

44.

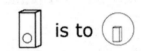

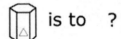

45. Simplify the following expression:

$3x^3 + 2x^2 + 5x - 7 + 4x^2 - 5x + 2 - 3x^3$

    a. $6x^2 - 9$
    b. $6x^2 - 5$
    c. $6x^2 - 10x - 5$
    d. $6x^2 + 10x - 9$

46. A building is 15 m long and 20 m wide and 10 m high. What is the volume of the building?

    a. 45 m³

    b. 3,000 m³

    c. 1500 m³

    d. 300 m³

47. What is 465,890 less 456,890?

    a. 9,000

    b. 7000

    c. 8970

    d. 8500

48. Solve 3/4 + 2/4 + 1.2

    a. 1 1/7

    b. 2 3/4

    c. 2 9/20

    d. 3 1/4

49. A map uses a scale of 1:2,000. How much distance on the ground is 5.2 inches on the map if the scale is in inches?

    a. 100,400

    b. 10, 500

    c. 10,440

    d. 10,400

50. A bag contains 38 black balls and 42 white balls. What is the ratio of black balls to white?

    a. 9:11

    b. 1:3

    c. 19:21

    d. 11:9

Section III – Science

1. A motorcycle travelling 90 mph accelerates to pass a truck. Five seconds later the car is going 120 mph. Calculate the motorcycles' acceleration

    a. 5 mph/second^2
    b. 10 mph/second^2
    c. 15 mph/second^2
    d. 20 mph/second^2

2. Which of the following disciplines have a close relationship with cell biology?

    a. Genetics
    b. Genealogy
    c. Paleontology
    d. Archaeology

3. A solution with a pH value of greater than 7 is

    a. Base
    b. Acid
    c. Neutral
    d. None of the above

4. Ohm's law states

    a. The voltage across a resistor is not equal to the product of the resistance and the current flowing through it.

    b. The voltage across a resistor is equal to the product of the resistance and the current flowing through it.

    c. The voltage across a resistor is greater than the product of the resistance.

    d. The voltage across a resistor is equal to the current flowing through it.

5. Which statement below regarding Eukaryotic and prokaryotic cells is correct?

    a. Both are organelles
    b. Eukaryotic are not organelles
    c. Both have DNA
    d. Both have single membrane compartments

6. Electricity is a general term encompassing a variety of phenomena resulting from the presence and flow of electric charge. Which of the following statements about electricity is/are true?

a. Electrically charged matter is influenced by, and produces, electromagnetic fields.

b. Electric current is a movement or flow of electrically charged particles.

c. Electric potential is a fundamental interaction between the magnetic field and the presence and motion of an electric charge.

d. An influence produced by an electric charge on other charges in its vicinity is an electric field.

7. Which of these is not a process involved in cellular biology?

a. Active transport

b. Adhesion

c. Subversion

d. Cell signaling

8. When we say that important traits for scientific classification are homologous, "homologous" means

a. Being shared among two or more animals with the same parent.

b. Being coincidentally shared by two totally different creatures.

c. Being inherited by the organisms' common ancestors.

d. Mutating beyond all reasonable expectations.

9. The manner in which instructions for building proteins, the basic structural molecules of living material are written in the DNA, is

a. Genotypic assignment

b. Chromosome pattern

c. Genetic code

d. Genetic fingerprinting

10. A _____ is a unit of inherited material, encoded by a strand of DNA and transcribed by RNA.

a. Allele

b. Phenotype

c. Gene

d. Genotype

11. A runner can sprint 6 meters per second. How far will she travel in 2 minutes?

   a. 600 meters
   b. 720 meters
   c. 760 meters
   d. 800 meters

12. Which of these is not an area studied in cell biology?

   a. Cells physiological properties
   b. Cell structure
   c. Cell life cycle
   d. Cellular scientists' biographies

13. Why is detection of pathogens complicated?

   a. They evolve so quickly
   b. They die so quickly
   c. They are invisible
   d. They multiply so quickly

14. Calculate the molarity of a sugar solution if 4 liters of the solution contains 8 moles of sugar?

   a. 0.5 M
   b. 8 M
   c. 2 M
   d. 80 M

15. Which of the following is/are not included in Ohm's Law?

   a. Ohm's Law defines the relationships between (P) power, (E) voltage, (I) current, and (R) resistance.

   b. One ohm is the resistance value through which one volt will maintain a current of one ampere.

   c. Using Ohm's Law, voltage is determined using V = IR, with I equaling current and R equaling resistance.

   d. An ohm (Ω) is a unit of electrical voltage.

16. How many elements are represented on the modern periodic table?

    a. 122 elements

    b. 99 elements

    c. 102 elements

    d. 118 elements

17. Which, if any, of the following statements are false?

    a. A mutation is a permanent change in the DNA sequence of a gene.

    b. Mutations in a gene's DNA sequence can alter the amino acid sequence of the protein encoded by the gene.

    c. Mutations in DNA sequences usually occur spontaneously.

    d. Mutations in DNA sequences can caused by exposure to environmental agents such as sunshine.

18. Three cars are travelling down an even road at a velocity of 110 m/s, calculate the car with the highest momentum if they are all moving at the same speed, but the first car weighs 2500 kg, second car weighs 2650 kg and third car weighs 2009 kg?

    a. First car

    b. Second car

    d. Third car

    d. All have same momentum

19. Starting with the weakest, arrange the fundamental forces of nature in order of strength.

    a. Gravity, Weak Nuclear Force, Electromagnetic Force, Strong Nuclear Force

    b. Weak Nuclear Force, Gravity, Electromagnetic Force, Strong Nuclear Force

    c. Strong Nuclear Force, Weak Nuclear Force, Electromagnetic Force, Gravity

    d. Gravity, Strong Nuclear Force, Weak Nuclear Force, Electromagnetic Force

20. What are electrons?

    a. Subatomic particles that carry a negative charge

    b. Subatomic particles that carry a positive charge

    c. Subatomic particles that carry both a negative and positive charge

    d. None of the above

21. Cell culture is defined as

a. The technique for growing cells independent of a living organism within the confines of a laboratory.

b. The process of killing cells through use of lasers.

c. The method of creating cellular communities.

d. A method for localizing proteins in tissue slices.

22. _____, which refers to the repeatability of measurement, does not require knowledge of the correct or true value.

a. Precision

b. Value

c. Certainty

d. Accuracy

23. How much force is needed to accelerate a car weighing 2,000 kg, at a rate of 3 m/s²?

a. 6000 N

b. 10,000 N

c. 4000 N

d. 8000 N

24. Describe the periodic table.

a. The periodic table is a tabular display of the chemical compounds organized on the basis of their atomic numbers, electron configurations, and recurring chemical properties.

b. The periodic table is a tabular display of the chemical elements, organized on the basis of their atomic numbers, electron configurations, and recurring chemical properties.

c. The periodic table is a tabular display of the chemical subatomic particles, organized on the basis of their atomic numbers, electron configurations, and recurring chemical properties.

d. None of the above.

25. The scientific discipline that studies the physiological aspects, structures, life cycles and division of cells is called _____.

    a. Physiology

    b. Cell science

    c. Biochemistry

    d. Cell biology

26. What is the minimum amount of energy required to remove an electron from an atom or ion in the gas phase?

    a. Ionization energy

    b. Valence energy

    c. Atomic energy

    d. Ionic energy

27. In a redox reaction, the number of electrons lost is

    a. Less than the number of electrons gained

    b. More than the number of electrons gained

    c. Equal to the number of electrons gained

    d. None of the above

28. In terms of the scientific method, the term _____ refers to the act of noticing or perceiving something and/or recording a fact or occurrence.

    a. Observation

    b. Diligence

    c. Perception

    d. Control

29. The _____ Theory defines acids and bases in terms of the electron-pair concept; according to its definition, an acid is an electron-pair acceptor, and a base is an electron-pair donor.

    a. Arrhenius

    b. Lewis

    c. Clark

    d. Brønstead-Lowry

30. What is the molarity of a solution containing 5 moles of solute in 250 milliliters of solution?

    a. 20 M

    b. 15 M

    c. 0.104 M

    d. 1.25 M

31. The property of a conductor that restricts its internal flow of electrons is:

    a. Friction

    b. Power

    c. Current

    d. Resistance

32. Describe bacteria.

    a. Prokaryotic microorganisms that are usually just a few micrometers long.

    b. A single-celled organism.

    c. A virus.

    d. Three or more molecules clumped together.

33. What is the difference, of any, between kinetic energy and potential energy?

    a. Kinetic energy is the energy of a body that results from heat while potential energy is the energy possessed by an object that is chilled.

    b. Kinetic energy is the energy of a body that results from motion while potential energy is the energy possessed by an object by virtue of its position or state, e.g., as in a compressed spring.

    c. There is no difference between kinetic and potential energy; all energy is the same.

    d. Potential energy is the energy of a body that results from motion while kinetic energy is the energy possessed by an object by virtue of its position or state, e.g., as in a compressed spring.

34. A rocket releases a satellite into orbit around Earth. The satellite travels at 2000 m/s in 25 seconds. What is the acceleration?

    a. 60 m/sec^2

    b. 80 m/sec^2

    c. 100 m/sec^2

    d. 120 m/sec^2

35. Name the four states in which matter exists.

    a. Concrete, liquid, gas, and plasma

    b. Solid, fluid, gas, and plasma

    c. Solid, liquid, vapor, and plasma

    d. Solid, liquid, gas, and plasma

36. Which one of the following best describes the function of a cell membrane?

    a. It controls the substances entering and leaving the cell.

    b. It keeps the cell in shape.

    c. It controls the substances entering the cell.

    d. It supports the cell structures

37. Describe electric current.

    a. Electric current is the flow of voltage

    b. Electric current is the movement of negative ions.

    c. Electric current is the flow of electric charge through a medium.

    d. None of the above

38. Which of the following is not a typical shape for a bacterium?

    a. Rod

    b. Spiral

    c. Sphere

    d. Cube

39. What is usually the result when acid reacts with most of the metals?

    a. Carbon dioxide

    b. Oxygen gas

    c. Nitrogen gas

    d. Hydrogen gas

40. Which of these is not a rank within the area of classification or taxonomy?

    a. Species

    b. Family

    c. Genus

    d. Relative position

41. Which of the following statements about the periodic table of the elements is true?

    a. On the periodic table, the elements are arranged according to their atomic mass.

    b. The way in which the elements are arranged allows for predictions to made about their behavior.

    c. The vertical columns of the table are called rows.

    d. The horizontal rows of the table are called groups.

42. The scientific term _____ refers to a practical test designed with the intention that its results be relevant to a particular theory or set of theories.

    a. Procedure

    b. Variable

    c. Hypothesis

    d. Experiment

43. Substances that deactivate catalysts are called

    a. Inhibitors

    b. Catalytic poisons

    c. Positive catalysts

    d. None of the above

44. What is the force per unit area exerted against a surface by the weight of air above that surface in the Earth's atmosphere?

    a. Gravitational force

    b. Atmospheric pressure

    c. Barometric density

    d. Aneroid pressure

45. Describe kinetic energy.

    a. Kinetic energy is the energy an object possesses due to its mass.

    b. Kinetic energy is the energy an object possesses due to its motion.

    c. Kinetic energy is the energy an object possesses due to its chemical properties.

    d. Kinetic energy is the stored energy an object possesses.

46. Another term for biological classification is:

 a. Darwinian classification

 b. Animal classification

 c. Molecular classification

 d. Scientific classification

47. When do oxidation and reduction reactions occur?

 a. One after the other

 b. In separate reactions

 c. On the product side of the reaction

 d. Simultaneously

48. What type of gene is not expressed as a trait unless inherited by both parents?

 a. Principal gene

 b. Latent gene

 c. Recessive gene

 d. Dominant gene

49. A _____ _____ is an approximation or simulation of a real system that omits all but the most essential variables of the system.

 a. Scientific method

 b. Independent variable

 c. Control group

 d. Scientific model

50. How many moles of Na are needed to make 4.5 liters of a 1.5 M Na solution?

 a. 3 mol

 b. 0.33 M

 c. 0.33 mol

 d. 3 M

51. Neutrons are necessary within an atomic nucleus because

 a. They bind with protons via nuclear force

 b. They bind with nuclei via nuclear force

 c. They bind with protons via electromagnetic force

d. They bind with nuclei via electromagnetic force

52. How do atoms of different elements combine to form chemical mixtures?

a. Atoms of different elements combine in simple whole-number ratios to form chemical compounds.

b. Atoms of different components combine in simple fractional ratios to form chemical compounds.

c. Atoms of the same element combine in simple whole-number ratios to form chemical compounds.

d. Atoms of different elements combine in simple whole-number ratios to form chemical mixtures.

53. Which of the following statements is false?

a. Most enzymes are proteins

b. Enzymes are catalysts

c. Most enzymes are inorganic

d. Enzymes are large biological molecules

54. _____ are compounds that contain hydrogen, can dissolve in water to release hydrogen ions into solution, and, in an aqueous solution, can conduct electricity.

a. Caustics

b. Bases

c. Acids

d. Salts

55. Find the momentum of a round stone weighing 12.05 kg rolling down a hill at 8 m/s.

a. 95 kg m/sec down the hill.

b. 96.4 kg m/sec down the hill.

c. 100 kg m/sec down the hill.

d. 90 kg m/sec down the hill.

56. Which of the following statements about non-metals are false?

a. A non-metal is a substance that conducts heat and electricity poorly.

b. The majority of the known chemical elements are non-metals.

c. A non-metal is brittle or waxy or gaseous.

d. None of the statements are false.

57. What is the name of the discipline that studies bacteria?

    a. Bacteriography

    b. Bacteriology

    c. Bacteriepathy

    d. Bacterioscopy

58. What are the basic structural units of nucleic acids (DNA or RNA) whose sequence determines individual hereditary characteristics?

    a. Gene

    b. Nucleotide

    c. Phosphate

    d. Nitrogen base

59. Which of these statements about light energy is/are true?

    a. Light consists of electromagnetic waves in the visible range.

    b. The fundamental particle or quantum of light is a photon.

    c. A and B are true.

    d. None of the statements are true.

60. List the classifications of organisms in order of size.

    a. Genus, Kingdom, Phylum/division, Class, Order, and Family Species

    b. Order, Kingdom, Phylum/division, Genus, Class, and Family Species

    c. Genus, Kingdom, Phylum/division, Class, Order, and Family Species

    d. Kingdom ,Genus, Phylum/division, Class, Order, and Family Species

    e. Family species, Order, Class, Phylum/division, Kingdom, and Genus

61. Explain chemical bonds.

    a. Chemical bonds are attractions between atoms that form chemical substances containing two or more atoms.

    b. Chemical bonds are attractions between protons that form chemical elements containing two or more atoms.

    c. Chemical bonds are two or more atoms that form chemical substances.

    d. None of the above

62. The number of protons in the nucleus of an atom is the

   a. Atomic mass.

   b. Atomic weight.

   c. Atomic number.

   d. None of the above.

63. The molarity of an aqueous solution of CaCl is defined as the

   a. moles of CaCl per milliliter of solution

   b. grams of CaCl per liter of water

   c. grams of CaCl per milliliter of solution

   d. moles of CaCl per liter of solution

64. An electron is:

   a. A tiny particle with a negative charge.

   b. A tiny particle with a positive charge.

   c. A tiny particle with a negative charge that orbits a nucleus.

   d. A tiny particle with a positive charge that orbits an atom.

65. What law states that, in a chemical change, energy can be neither created nor destroyed, but only changed from one form to another?

   a. The Law of the Preservation of Matter

   b. The Law of the Conservation of Energy

   c. The Law of the Conservation of Energy

   d. The Law of the Conservation of Energy

66. What is the simplest unit of any compound?

   a. Atom

   b. Proton

   c. Molecule

   d. Compound

67. Sex chromosomes are designated as being "X" or "Y" chromosomes. In terms of sex chromosomes, what differences exist between males and females?

a. Females have two X chromosomes and males have one X chromosome and one Y chromosome.

b. Females have one X chromosome, and males have one X chromosome and one Y chromosome.

c. Females have one Y chromosome, while males have one X chromosome.

d. Females have one X chromosome and one Y chromosome, and males have two X chromosomes.

68. A biofilm is

a. A dense aggregation of bacteria attached to surfaces.

b. A type of bacteria which causes disease.

c. A cluster of bacteria which is healthy to consume.

d. Bacteria which aids in digestion.

69. Identify the chemical properties of water.

a. Water has two hydrogen atoms covalently bonded to one oxygen atom.

b. Water has two oxygen atoms covalently bonded to one hydrogen atom.

c. Water has two hydrogen atoms polar covalently bonded to one oxygen atom.

d. Water has two oxygen atoms polar covalently bonded to one hydrogen atom.

70. Which of the following is not true of atomic theory?

a. Originated in the early 19th century with the work of John Dalton.

b. Is the field of physics that describes the characteristics and properties of atoms that make up matter.

c. Explains temperature as the momentum of atoms.

d. Explains macroscopic phenomenon through the behavior of microscopic atoms.

71. Calculate the molarity of 2.5 liters of a lithium fluoride, LiF solution that contains 52 grams of LiF. (Gram-formula - atomic mass =26 grams/mole)

a. 0.8 M

b. 1.5 M

c. 0.5 mol

d. 2 mol

72. In physics, _____ is the force that opposes the relative motion of two bodies in contact.

     a. Resistance

     b. Abrasiveness

     c. Friction

     d. Antagonism

73. What is the difference between anabolism and catabolism?

     a. Anabolism is the series of chemical reactions resulting in the synthesis of inorganic compounds, and catabolism is a series of chemical reactions that break down larger molecules.

     b. Anabolism is the series of chemical reactions resulting in the synthesis of organic compounds, and catabolism is a series of chemical reactions that combine larger molecules.

     c. Catabolism is the series of chemical reactions resulting in the synthesis of organic compounds, and anabolism is a series of chemical reactions that break down larger molecules.

     d. Anabolism is the series of chemical reactions resulting in the synthesis of organic compounds, and catabolism is a series of chemical reactions that break down larger molecules.

74. What results when acid reacts with a base?

     a. A weak acid

     b. A weak base

     c. A salt and water

     d. Hydrogen

75. What is a reaction where an element gains electrons is known as?

     a. Reduction

     b. Oxidation

     c. Sublimation

     d. Condensation

Answer Key

Section 1 – Verbal Ability

1. B
We can infer from this passage that sickness from an infectious disease can be easily transmitted from one person to another.

From the passage, "Infectious pathologies are also called communicable diseases or transmissible diseases, due to their potential of transmission from one person or species to another by a replicating agent (as opposed to a toxin)."

2. A
Two other names for infectious pathologies are communicable diseases and transmissible diseases.

From the passage, "Infectious pathologies are also called communicable diseases or transmissible diseases, due to their potential of transmission from one person or species to another by a replicating agent (as opposed to a toxin)."

3. C
Infectivity describes the ability of an organism to enter, survive and multiply in the host. This is taken directly from the passage, and is a definition type question.

Definition type questions can be answered quickly and easily by scanning the passage for the word you are asked to define.

"Infectivity" is an unusual word, so it is quick and easy to scan the passage looking for this word.

4. B
We know an infection is not synonymous with an infectious disease because an infection may not cause important clinical symptoms or impair host function.

5. C
We can infer from the passage that, a virus is too small to be seen with the naked eye. Clearly, if they are too small to be seen with a microscope, then they are too small to be seen with the naked eye.

6. D
Viruses infect all types of organisms. This is taken directly from the passage, "Viruses infect all types of organisms, from animals and plants to bacteria and single-celled organisms."

7. C
The passage does not say exactly how many parts prions and viroids consist of. It does say, "Unlike prions and viroids, viruses consist of two or three parts ..." so we can infer they consist of either less than two or more than three parts.

8. B
A common virus spread by coughing and sneezing is Influenza.

9. C
The cumulus stage of a thunderstorm is the beginning of the thunderstorm.

This is taken directly from the passage, "The first stage of a thunderstorm is the cumulus, or developing stage."

10. D
The passage lists four ways that air is heated. One of the ways is, heat created by water vapor condensing into liquid.

11. A
The sequence of events can be taken from these sentences:

As the moisture carried by the [1] air currents rises, it rapidly cools into liquid drops of water, which appear as cumulus clouds. As the water vapor condenses into liquid, it [2] releases heat, which warms the air. This in turn causes the air to become less dense than the surrounding dry air and [3] rise further.

12. C
The purpose of this text is to explain when meteorologists consider a thunderstorm severe.

The main idea is the first sentence, "The United States National Weather Service classifies thunderstorms as severe when they reach a predetermined level." After the first sentence, the passage explains and elaborates on this idea. Everything is this passage is related to this idea, and there are no other major ideas in this passage that are central to the whole passage.

13. A
From this passage, we can infer that different areas and countries have different criteria for determining a severe storm.

From the passage we can see that most of the US has a criteria of, winds over 50 knots (58 mph or 93 km/h), and hail ¾ inch (2 cm). For the Central US, hail must be 1 inch (2.5 cm) in diameter. In Canada, winds must be 90 km/h or greater, hail 2 centimeters in diameter or greater, and rainfall more than 50 millimeters in 1 hour, or 75 millimeters in 3 hours.

Option D is incorrect because the Canadian system is the same for hail, 2 centimeters in diameter.

14. C
With hail above the minimum size of 2.5 cm. diameter, the Central Region of the United States National Weather Service would issue a severe thunderstorm warning.

15. D
Clouds in space are made of different materials attracted by gravity. Clouds on Earth are made of water droplets or ice crystals.

Choice D is the best answer. Notice also that Choice D is the most specific.

16. C
The main idea is the first sentence of the passage; a cloud is a visible mass of droplets or frozen crystals floating in the atmosphere above the surface of the Earth or other planetary body.

The main idea is very often the first sentence of the paragraph.

17. C
Nephology, which is the study of cloud physics.

18. C
This question asks about the process, and gives options that can be confirmed or eliminated easily.

From the passage, "Dense, deep clouds reflect most light, so they appear white, at least from the top. Cloud droplets scatter light very efficiently, so the further into a cloud light travels, the weaker it gets. This accounts for the gray or dark appearance at the base of large clouds."

We can eliminate choice A, since water droplets inside the cloud do not reflect light is false.

We can eliminate choice B, since, water droplets outside the cloud reflect light, it appears dark, is false.

Choice C is correct.

19. A
The correct order of ingredients is brown sugar, baking soda and chocolate chips.

20. B
Sturdy: strong, solid in structure or person. In context, Stir in chocolate chips by hand with a *sturdy* wooden spoon.

21. A
Disperse: to scatter in different directions or break up. In context, Stir until the chocolate chips and nuts are evenly *dispersed.*

22. B
You can stop stirring the nuts when they are evenly distributed. From the passage, "Stir until the chocolate chips and nuts are evenly dispersed."

23. A
Larvae spend most of their time in search of food and their food is leaves.

24. B
From the passage, the ants provide some degree of protection

25. C
The association is mutual so both benefit.

26. A
Navy SEALS are the maritime component of the United States Special Operations Command (USSOCOM).

27. C
Working underwater separates SEALs from other military units. This is taken directly from the passage.

28. D
SEALs also belong to the Navy and the Coast Guard.

29. A
The CIA also participated. From the passage, the raid was conducted by a "team of 40 *CIA-led* Navy SEALS."

30. C
From the passage, "The Navy SEALs were part of the Naval Special Warfare Development Group, previously called "Team 6". "

31. B
This question is taken directly from the passage.

32. A
The Egyptians believed gods loved gardens.

33. B
Cypresses and palms were the most popular trees in Assyrian Gardens.

34. B
Vegetable gardens came before ornamental gardens.

The earliest forms of gardens emerged from the people's need to grow herbs and vegetables. It was only later that rich individuals created gardens for the purely decorative purpose.

35. A
The ancient Roman gardens are known by their statues and sculptures ...

36. D
After the fall of Rome, gardening was only for medicinal purposes, AND gardening declined in the Middle Ages, so we can infer gardening declined after the fall of Rome.

37. C
From the passage, "After the fall of Rome gardening was only done with the purpose of growing medicinal herbs and decorating church altars," so Choice C.

38. B
From the passage, "Mosaics and glazed tiles used to decorate elaborate fountains are specific to Islamic gardens."

39. B
From the passage, "Often called "rainforests of the sea", coral reefs form some of the most diverse ecosystems on Earth."

40. A
Read the passage carefully – "The polyps are like tiny sea anemones, to which they are closely related."

41. C
This question is designed to confuse by giving variation of the same information. Read the passage carefully for the correct answer.

42. D
This question is designed to confuse by giving variation of the same information. Read the passage carefully for the correct answer.

Verbal Ability Part II - Vocabulary

43. C
Dauntless: adj. Invulnerable to fear or intimidation.

44. A
Juxtaposed: adj. Placed side by side often for comparison or contrast.

45. B
Regicide: v. killing of a king.

46. A
Pernicious: adj. Causing much harm in a subtle way.

47. A
Immune: adj. Resistant to a particular infection or toxin owing to the presence of specific antibodies.

48. B
Nimble: adj. Quick and light in movement or action.

49. A
Queries: n. Questions or inquiries.

50. C
Depose: To remove (a leader) from (high) office, without killing the incumbent.

51. D
Pedestrian: Ordinary, dull; everyday; unexceptional.

52. B
Petulant: adj. Childishly irritable.

53. D
Pesticide: n. A substance used for destroying insects or other organisms harmful to cultivated plants or to animals.

54. D
Salient: adj. worthy or note or relevant.

55. B
Sedentary: adj. not moving or sitting in one place.

56. A
Famine: n. extreme scarcity of food.

57. A
Stint: n. To be sparing.

58. A
Precipitate: v. to rain.

59. C
Edify: v. To instruct or improve morally or intellectually.

60. B
Egress: n. An exit or way out.

61. A
Recede: v. To move back, to move away.

62. A
Confidential: adj. kept secret within a certain circle of persons; not intended to be known publicly.

63. A
Aggravate: v. to make worse, or more severe; to render less tolerable or less excusable; to make more offensive; to enhance; to intensify.

64. B
Debut: n. a performer's first-time performance to the public.

65. B
Hormones: n. A regulatory substance produced in an organism and transported in tissue fluids such as blood or sap to stimulate specific cells.

66. B
Importune: v. To harass with persistent requests.

67. B
Sedulous: adj. Showing dedication and diligence.

68. A
Tincture: n. alcoholic drink with plant extracts used for medicine.

69. C
Felony: n. Serious criminal offence that is punishable by death or imprisonment above a year.

70. A
Bibliophile: n. One who loves books.

71. A
Monsoons: n. The rainy season accompanying the wet monsoon.

72. D
Volatile: adj. Explosive.

73. B
Plaintive: adj. Sorrowful, mournful or melancholic.

74. B
Truism: n. Self evident or clear obvious truth.

75. B
Foment: v. to encourage or incite troublesome acts.

76. A
Funereal: Adj. dignified, solemn that is appropriate for a funeral.

77. A
Flagrant: obvious and offensive, blatant, scandalous.

78. B
Moss

79. A
Nexus: n. A connection or series of connections linking two or more things.

80. A
Zealot: n. A person who is very passionate and fanatic about his specific objectives or beliefs.

Section II – Mathematics

1. A
$1/3 \times 3/4 = 3/12 = 1/4$

2. D
$75/1500 = 15/300 = 3/60 = 1/20$

3. B
$-4x^2 + x + 5$
$(-3x^2 + 2x + 6) + (-x^2 - x - 1)$
$-3x^2 + 2x + 6 - x^2 - x - 1$
$-4x^2 + x + 5$

4. D
$3.14 + 2.73 = 5.87$ and $5.87 + 23.7 = 29.57$

5. D
First add all the numbers $200,000 + 10,020 + 30,000 + 15,000 + 1080 = 256,100$. Then divide by 5 (the number of data provided) $= 256,100/5 = 51,220$

6. C
0.27 + 0.33 = 0.6 = 60/100 = 3/5.

7. D
3.13 + 7.87 = 11 and 11 X 5 = 55

8. A
3 x 3 x 3 x 3 = 81

9. B
2/4 X 3/4 = 6/16, in lowest terms = 3/8

10. D
$2(5)^3 - (2)^3$ = 2(125) − 8 = 250 − 8 = 242

11. C
3/10 * 90 = 3 * 90/10 = 270/10 = 27

12. C
First add all the numbers 1 + 2 + 3 + 4 + 5 +6 + 7 +8 + 9 + 10 = 55. Then divide by 10 (the number of data provided) = 55/5 = 11

13. B
.4/100 * 36 = .4 * 36/100 = 14.4/100 = 0.144

14. D
To solve for x,
5x − 7x + 3 = -1
5x − 7x = -1 -3
-2x = -4
x = -4/ -2
x = 2

15. B
The numbers are 15 and 6.
x + 7 = 21 => x = 21 -7
$x^2 + y^2 = 261$

$(21 - 7)^2 + y^2 = 261$
$441 - 42y + y^2 + y^2 = 261$
$2y^2 - 42y + 180 = 0$
$y^2 - 21y + 90 = 0$
$y_{1,2} = 21 \pm \sqrt{441 - 360}/2$
$y_{1,2} = 21 \pm \sqrt{81}/2$
$y_{1,2} = 21 \pm 9/2$
$y_1 = 15$
$y_2 = 6$

$x_1 = 21 = y_1 = 21 - 15 = 6$
$x_2 = 21 - y_2 = 21 - 6 = 15$

16. C
To solve for x, first simplify the equation
5x + 2x + 14 = 14x − 7
7x + 14 = 14x -7
7x − 14x + 14 = -7
7x − 14x = -7 − 14
-7x = -21
x = -21/-7
x=3

17. C
5z + 5 = 3z +6 + 11
5z -3z + 5 =6 + 11
5z − 3z = 6 + 11 -5
2z = 17 − 5
2z = 12
z= 12/2
z= 6

18. C
To make this easier we can break 81 to be 9 x 9 and then find the prime factors of each of these prime numbers. The prime factors of 9 = 3 x 3 and the prime factors of 9 = 3 x 3 Prime factors of 81 = 3 x 3 x 3 x 3

19. D
Price increased by $5 ($25-$20). The percent increase is 5/20 x 100 = 5 x 5=25%

20. D
30/100 x 150 = 3 x 15 = 45 (increase in number of correct answers). So the number of correct answers in second test will be the number of correct answers in the first test plus the increase, which is, 150 + 45 = 195

21. C
(4 x 4 x 4) + (2 x 2 x 2 x 2) = 64 + 16 = 80

22. D
As the lawn is square, the length of one side will be = $\sqrt{62500}$ = 250 meters. So

the perimeters will be: 250 × 4 = 1000 meters.
The total cost will be 1000 × $5.5 = $5500.

23. C
p = 1.5 x 18 = 27 kg x m/s into the field.

24. D
The decimal point moves 2 spaces right to be placed after 2, which is the first non-zero number. Thus it is 2.04×10^2

25. B
There are 50 balls in the basket now. Let x be the number of yellow balls that are to be added to make 65%. So the equation becomes
X + 15 /X + 50 = 65/100
X = 50

26. C
There are 144 students and each bus holds 36, so 144/36 = 4 buses.

27. D
-2

$$x^2 + 4x + 4 = 0$$
$$x^2 + 2x + 2x + 4 = 0$$
$$x(x+2) + 2(x+2) = 0$$
$$(x+2)(x+2) = 0$$
$$(x+2)^2 = 0$$
$$x = -2$$

28. C
The sum of angles around a point is 360°
d+300 = 360°
d = 60°

29. A
Diameter = 2 x radius.
Circumference = π x Diameter

Distance(meters) = (Circumference x Revolutions)/100

Distance(meters) = [((25 x 2) π) x 175]/100
Distance(meters) = 8750 π/100
Distance = 87.5 π m

30. C
Pythagorean Theorem:
(Hypotenuse)² = (Perpendicular)² + (Base)²
$h^2 = a^2 + b^2$

Given: $a^2 + b^2 = 25$
$h^2 = 25$
h = 5

31. D
Shaded area= Outer area – Inner area(square + rectangle)
Shaded area= (8 x 8) –{(2 x 2) + [(3 + 2) x 4]}, = 64 – (4 + 20), =
64- 24
Shaded area= 40 cm²

32. A
Black stone for 200 tiles = 200 x [Total tile area – Inner white area(4 triangles)]
= 200 x [(162)-(4x1/2 x 8 x 8)] = 200 x (256-128) = 200 x 128 = 25600 cm²
Converting to meters – 1 cm. = 0.01 meters
= 25600/100 m²
= 256 m²

33. B
Slope (m) = change in y/change in x

(x^1, y^1)=(-1,2) & (x^2, y^2)= (-4,-4)
Slope = (-4 – 2)/[-4-(-1)]= -6/-3
Slope =2

34. A
The equation for the total liters of wine will be y = 0.20x + 2

35. C
If it takes 12 men to operate four machines, then, 12 is to 4, as X is to 20. So X must be 3 X 20 = 60.

36. C
If there are 5 friends and each drink costs

$1.89, we can round up to $2 per drink and estimate the total cost at, 5 X $2 = $10.

The actual cost is 5 X $1.89 = $9.45.

37. D
First convert 500g to kg = 500/1000 = 0.5kg, momentum = 0.5 x 3.5 = 1.75 kg x m/s along the road

38. A
$\sqrt{121}$

39. D
The smallest prime number that can divide 25 is 5. 25/5 = 5. Prime factors of 25 = 5 x 5

40. D
The decimal point moves 5 places left to be placed after 2, which is the first non-zero number. Thus its 2.011×10^{-5} The answer is in the negative because the decimal

moved left

41. D
7: 25 =X:100
25/7 = 3.5
100/3.5 = 28.5

42. B
The relation is two upright figures in the first set, and 2 horizontal figures in the second set.

43. C
The first pair contains a box with a circle inside, and the same figure on its side.

44. C
The inside and larger shapes are reversed.

45. B
$6x^2 - 5$
$3x^3 + 2x^2 + 5x - 7 + 4x^2 - 5x + 2 - 3x^3 = 6x^2 - 5$

46. B
Formula for volume of a shape is L x W x H = 15 x 20 x 10 = 3,000m³

47. A
465,890 - 456,890 = 9,000

48. C
3/4 + 2/4 + 1.2, first convert the decimal to fraction, = 3/4 + 2/4 + 1 1/5 = ¾ + 2/4 + 6/5 = (find common denominator) (15 + 10 + 24)/20 = 49/20 = 2 9/20

49. C
1 inch on map = 2,000 inches on ground. So 5.2 inches on map = 5.2 x 2,000 = 10,440 inches on ground.

50. C
The ratio of black balls to white is 38:42. Reduce to lowest terms = 19:21

Section III – Science

1. A
The formula for acceleration = A = $(V_f - V_0)/t$
so A = (120 -90)/5 sec = 5 mph/second²

2. A
Only genetics pertains directly to the cell's function. In the case of genetics, the cell of a new organism acquires traits of ancestral organisms.

3. A
A solution with a pH value of greater than 7 is base.

4. B
The voltage across a resistor is equal to the product of the resistance and the current flowing through it.

5. A
Eukaryotic and prokaryotic cells are both organelles.

6. C

Electric potential is a fundamental interaction between the magnetic field and the presence and motion of an electric charge.

Electric potential is the capacity of an electric field to do work on an electric charge, typically measured in volts, while electromagnetism is a fundamental interaction between the magnetic field and the presence and motion of an electric charge.

7. C

Subversion. Active transport, adhesion and cell signaling are all involved in cellular biology.

8. C

Homologous is being inherited by the organisms' common ancestors. An example would be feathers and hair—both of which were structures that shared a common ancestral trait.

9. C

The manner in which instructions for building proteins, the basic structural molecules of living material are written in the DNA is a **genetic code**.

10. C

A gene is a unit of inherited material, encoded by a strand of DNA and transcribed by RNA.

11. B

Speed = (total distance traveled)/(total time taken)
6 = x/120   (convert minutes to seconds)
6 * 120 = x
X = 720 meters

12. D

Cellular scientists' biographies are not studied in cell biology. The physiological properties of cells, cell structure and the life cycle of a cell are all valid topics of study within the field of cell biology.

13. A

Detection of pathogens can be complicated because they evolve so quickly.

14. C

Molarity = moles of solute/liters of solu-

tion = 8/4 = 2

15. D

An ohm (Ω) is a unit of electrical voltage is not true.

Note: An ohm is a unit of electrical resistance.

16. D

The periodic table as it is now contains 118 elements.

17. C

Mutations in DNA sequences usually occur spontaneously is false.

18. C

Momentum is a product of velocity and mass. If they are all traveling at the same speed, the car that weighs the most would have the highest momentum.

19. A

Starting with the weakest, the fundamental forces of nature in order of strength are, Gravity, Weak nuclear force, Electromagnetic force, Strong nuclear force.

20. A

Electrons are subatomic particles that carry a negative charge.

21. A

Cell culture is the technique for growing cells independent of a living organism within the confines of a laboratory. The cell culture is generally grown in a test-tube environment or on a petri dish.

22. A

Precision, which refers to the repeatability of measurement, does not require knowledge of the correct or true value.

23. A

Force = Mass times Acceleration Measured in Newtons.
F = 2000 kg X 3 m/sec^2 = 6000 N

24. B
The periodic table is a tabular display of the chemical elements, organized on the basis of their atomic numbers, electron configurations, and recurring chemical properties.

25. D
The scientific discipline that studies the physiological aspects, structures, life cycles and division of cells is called cell biology.

26. A
Ionization energy is the minimum amount of energy required to remove an electron from an atom or ion in the gas phase.

27. C
Redox is a complete reaction comprising oxidation and reduction reactions that are each only half of the complete reaction. The same exact electrons lost in oxidation are what are gained in reduction.

28. A
In terms of the scientific method, the term **observation** refers to the act of noticing or perceiving something and/or recording a fact or occurrence.

29. B
The Lewis Theory defines acids and bases in terms of the electron-pair concept; according to its definition, an acid is an electron-pair acceptor, and a base is an electron-pair donor.

30. A
First convert 250 ml to liters, 250/1000 = 0.25 then calculate molarity = 5 moles/ 0.25 liters = 20 M.

31. D
The property of a conductor that restricts its internal flow of electrons is resistance.

32. A
Prokaryotic microorganisms that are usually just a few micrometers long.

33. B

Kinetic energy is the energy of a body that results from motion while potential energy is the energy possessed by an object by virtue of its position or state, e.g., as in a compressed spring.

34. B
The formula for acceleration $= A = (V_f - V_0)/t$
so $A = (2000 - 0)/25 \text{ sec} = 80 \text{ m/sec}^2$

35. A
The four states in which matter exists are solid, fluid, gas, and plasma.

The state of matter is determined by the strength of the bonds between the atoms that make up matter.

36. A
The cell membrane is a biological membrane that separates the interior of all cells from the outside environment. The cell membrane is selectively permeable to ions and organic molecules and controls the movement of substances in and out of cells.

37. C
Electric current is the flow of electric charge through a medium.

38. D
Cubes rarely occur naturally, especially in the micro world outside of the human eye. True cubes are usually deliberately created.

39. D
All acids contain hydrogen. When acids react with most metals, the metals displace the hydrogen and hydrogen gas is produced.

40. D
Relative position. Ranks include Domain, Kingdom, Phylum, Class, Order, Family, Genus, and Species.

41. B

The following statements about the periodic table of the elements is true,
The way in which the elements are arranged allows for predictions to made about their behavior.

42. D
The scientific term **experiment** refers to a practical test designed with the intention that its results be relevant to a particular theory or set of theories.

43. B
Substances that deactivate catalysts are called catalytic poisons.

44. B
Atmospheric pressure is the force per unit area exerted against a surface by the weight of air above that surface in the Earth's atmosphere.

45. B
Kinetic energy is the energy an object possesses due to its motion.

46. D
Scientific classification. The two phrases are interchangeable, although the former seems to more accurately reflect the purpose of classification: to categorize biological units.

47. D
Oxidation and reduction reactions are each just half of a redox reaction and both occur simultaneously, because the exact electrons lost in oxidation is what is gained in reduction.

48. C
A recessive gene is not expressed as a trait unless inherited by both parents.

49. D
A **scientific model** is an approximation or simulation of a real system that omits all but the most essential variables of the system.

50. A
$X/4.5 = 1.5$, $X = 4.5/1.5 = 3$ mol.

51. A
Neutrons are necessary within an atomic nucleus as they bind with protons via the nuclear force.

52. A
Atoms of different elements combine in simple whole-number ratios to form chemical compounds.

53. C
The following statement is false - Most enzymes are inorganic.

54. C
Acids are compounds that contain hydrogen and can dissolve in water to release hydrogen ions into solution.

55. B
Formula - P= kg x m/s
= 12.05kg x 8m/s
= 96.4 kg x m/s down the hill.

Note that the final answer has the proper SI unit of momentum (kg x m/s) after it and it also mentions the direction of the movement.

56. D
All of the statements are true.

a. A non-metal is a substance that conducts heat and electricity poorly.

b. The majority of the known chemical elements are non-metals.

c. A non-metal is brittle or waxy or gaseous.

57. B

The discipline that studies bacteria is Bacteriology.

58. A
Genes determine individual hereditary characteristics.

59. C
A and B are true.

      a. Light consists of electromagnetic waves in the visible range.
      b. The fundamental particle or quantum of light is a photon.

Note: Light energy is the only visible form of energy. A light bulb is a device that uses electrical energy to create electromagnetic energy in the form (in part) of visible light and heat.

60. A
The groups into which organisms are classified are called taxa and include, in order of size, Genus, Kingdom, Phylum/division, Class, Order, and Family Species.

61. A
Chemical bonds are attractions between atoms that form chemical substances containing two or more atoms.

62. C
In chemistry, the number of protons in the nucleus of an atom is known as the atomic number, which determines the chemical element to which the atom belongs.

63. D
The molarity of an aqueous solution of CaCl is defined as the moles of CaCl per liter of solution.

64. C
An electron is a tiny particle with a negative charge that orbits a nucleus.

65. C
The Law of the Conservation of Energy states that, in a chemical change, energy can be neither created nor destroyed, but only changed from one form to another.

66. A
An atom is the basic or fundamental unit of any matter or element.

67. A
Females have two X chromosomes and males have one X chromosome and one Y chromosome.

68. A
A biofilm is a dense aggregation of bacteria attached to surfaces. The density of these bacteria is based on many factors, such as environment, temperature, and how long they're left there undisturbed.

69. A
Water has two hydrogen atoms covalently bonded to one oxygen atom.

70. C
Choice C (Atomic theory explains temperature as the momentum of atoms.) is incorrect because atomic theory explains temperature as the motion of atoms (faster = hotter), not the momentum. The momentum of atoms explains the outward pressure that they exert.

71. A
First convert LiF grams to moles = 52 x 1/26 = 2. Now Molarity = 2 moles/2.5 liters = 0.8 M

72. C
In physics, friction is the force that opposes the relative motion of two bodies in contact.

73. D
Anabolism is the series of chemical reactions resulting in the synthesis of organic compounds, and catabolism is a series of chemical reactions that break down larger molecules.

74. C

When an acid and a base react, they neutralize each other's properties to form salt and water.

75. A

Reduction is a reaction that usually involves the gain of electrons that were lost in an oxidation reaction.

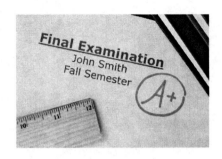

Practice Test Questions Set 2

The questions below are not exactly the same as you will find on the PAX RN - that would be too easy! And nobody knows what the questions will be and they change all the time. Below are general questions that cover the same subject areas as the PAX RN. So while the format and exact wording of the questions may differ slightly, and change from year to year, if you can answer the questions below, you will have no problem with the PAX RN.

For the best results, take this Practice Test as if it were the real exam. Set aside time when you will not be disturbed, and a location that is quiet and free of distractions. Read the instructions carefully, read each question carefully, and answer to the best of your ability.

Use the bubble answer sheets provided. When you have completed the Practice Test, check your answer against the Answer Key and read the explanation provided.

Do not attempt more than one set of practice test questions in one day. After completing the first practice test, wait two or three days before attempting the second set of questions.

Section I – Verbal Ability
Questions: 80 **Time:** 60 Minutes

Section II – Mathematics
Questions: 50 **Time:** 60 Minutes

Section III – Science
Questions: 75 **Time:** 60 minutes

Answer Sheet – Verbal Ability

1. (A) (B) (C) (D)   21. (A) (B) (C) (D)   41. (A) (B) (C) (D)   61. (A) (B) (C) (D)

2. (A) (B) (C) (D)   22. (A) (B) (C) (D)   42. (A) (B) (C) (D)   62. (A) (B) (C) (D)

3. (A) (B) (C) (D)   23. (A) (B) (C) (D)   43. (A) (B) (C) (D)   63. (A) (B) (C) (D)

4. (A) (B) (C) (D)   24. (A) (B) (C) (D)   44. (A) (B) (C) (D)   64. (A) (B) (C) (D)

5. (A) (B) (C) (D)   25. (A) (B) (C) (D)   45. (A) (B) (C) (D)   65. (A) (B) (C) (D)

6. (A) (B) (C) (D)   26. (A) (B) (C) (D)   46. (A) (B) (C) (D)   66. (A) (B) (C) (D)

7. (A) (B) (C) (D)   27. (A) (B) (C) (D)   47. (A) (B) (C) (D)   67. (A) (B) (C) (D)

8. (A) (B) (C) (D)   28. (A) (B) (C) (D)   48. (A) (B) (C) (D)   68. (A) (B) (C) (D)

9. (A) (B) (C) (D)   29. (A) (B) (C) (D)   49. (A) (B) (C) (D)   69. (A) (B) (C) (D)

10. (A) (B) (C) (D)   30. (A) (B) (C) (D)   50. (A) (B) (C) (D)   70. (A) (B) (C) (D)

11. (A) (B) (C) (D)   31. (A) (B) (C) (D)   51. (A) (B) (C) (D)   71. (A) (B) (C) (D)

12. (A) (B) (C) (D)   32. (A) (B) (C) (D)   52. (A) (B) (C) (D)   72. (A) (B) (C) (D)

13. (A) (B) (C) (D)   33. (A) (B) (C) (D)   53. (A) (B) (C) (D)   73. (A) (B) (C) (D)

14. (A) (B) (C) (D)   34. (A) (B) (C) (D)   54. (A) (B) (C) (D)   74. (A) (B) (C) (D)

15. (A) (B) (C) (D)   35. (A) (B) (C) (D)   55. (A) (B) (C) (D)   75. (A) (B) (C) (D)

16. (A) (B) (C) (D)   36. (A) (B) (C) (D)   56. (A) (B) (C) (D)   76. (A) (B) (C) (D)

17. (A) (B) (C) (D)   37. (A) (B) (C) (D)   57. (A) (B) (C) (D)   77. (A) (B) (C) (D)

18. (A) (B) (C) (D)   38. (A) (B) (C) (D)   58. (A) (B) (C) (D)   78. (A) (B) (C) (D)

19. (A) (B) (C) (D)   39. (A) (B) (C) (D)   59. (A) (B) (C) (D)   79. (A) (B) (C) (D)

20. (A) (B) (C) (D)   40. (A) (B) (C) (D)   60. (A) (B) (C) (D)   80. (A) (B) (C) (D)

Answer Sheet – Mathematics

1. Ⓐ Ⓑ Ⓒ Ⓓ	18. Ⓐ Ⓑ Ⓒ Ⓓ	35. Ⓐ Ⓑ Ⓒ Ⓓ
2. Ⓐ Ⓑ Ⓒ Ⓓ	19. Ⓐ Ⓑ Ⓒ Ⓓ	36. Ⓐ Ⓑ Ⓒ Ⓓ
3. Ⓐ Ⓑ Ⓒ Ⓓ	20. Ⓐ Ⓑ Ⓒ Ⓓ	37. Ⓐ Ⓑ Ⓒ Ⓓ
4. Ⓐ Ⓑ Ⓒ Ⓓ	21. Ⓐ Ⓑ Ⓒ Ⓓ	38. Ⓐ Ⓑ Ⓒ Ⓓ
5. Ⓐ Ⓑ Ⓒ Ⓓ	22. Ⓐ Ⓑ Ⓒ Ⓓ	39. Ⓐ Ⓑ Ⓒ Ⓓ
6. Ⓐ Ⓑ Ⓒ Ⓓ	23. Ⓐ Ⓑ Ⓒ Ⓓ	40. Ⓐ Ⓑ Ⓒ Ⓓ
7. Ⓐ Ⓑ Ⓒ Ⓓ	24. Ⓐ Ⓑ Ⓒ Ⓓ	41. Ⓐ Ⓑ Ⓒ Ⓓ
8. Ⓐ Ⓑ Ⓒ Ⓓ	25. Ⓐ Ⓑ Ⓒ Ⓓ	42. Ⓐ Ⓑ Ⓒ Ⓓ
9. Ⓐ Ⓑ Ⓒ Ⓓ	26. Ⓐ Ⓑ Ⓒ Ⓓ	43. Ⓐ Ⓑ Ⓒ Ⓓ
10. Ⓐ Ⓑ Ⓒ Ⓓ	27. Ⓐ Ⓑ Ⓒ Ⓓ	44. Ⓐ Ⓑ Ⓒ Ⓓ
11. Ⓐ Ⓑ Ⓒ Ⓓ	28. Ⓐ Ⓑ Ⓒ Ⓓ	45. Ⓐ Ⓑ Ⓒ Ⓓ
12. Ⓐ Ⓑ Ⓒ Ⓓ	29. Ⓐ Ⓑ Ⓒ Ⓓ	46. Ⓐ Ⓑ Ⓒ Ⓓ
13. Ⓐ Ⓑ Ⓒ Ⓓ	30. Ⓐ Ⓑ Ⓒ Ⓓ	47. Ⓐ Ⓑ Ⓒ Ⓓ
14. Ⓐ Ⓑ Ⓒ Ⓓ	31. Ⓐ Ⓑ Ⓒ Ⓓ	48. Ⓐ Ⓑ Ⓒ Ⓓ
15. Ⓐ Ⓑ Ⓒ Ⓓ	32. Ⓐ Ⓑ Ⓒ Ⓓ	49. Ⓐ Ⓑ Ⓒ Ⓓ
16. Ⓐ Ⓑ Ⓒ Ⓓ	33. Ⓐ Ⓑ Ⓒ Ⓓ	50. Ⓐ Ⓑ Ⓒ Ⓓ
17. Ⓐ Ⓑ Ⓒ Ⓓ	34. Ⓐ Ⓑ Ⓒ Ⓓ	

Answer Sheet – Science

1. (A) (B) (C) (D)	21. (A) (B) (C) (D)	41. (A) (B) (C) (D)	61. (A) (B) (C) (D)
2. (A) (B) (C) (D)	22. (A) (B) (C) (D)	42. (A) (B) (C) (D)	62. (A) (B) (C) (D)
3. (A) (B) (C) (D)	23. (A) (B) (C) (D)	43. (A) (B) (C) (D)	63. (A) (B) (C) (D)
4. (A) (B) (C) (D)	24. (A) (B) (C) (D)	44. (A) (B) (C) (D)	64. (A) (B) (C) (D)
5. (A) (B) (C) (D)	25. (A) (B) (C) (D)	45. (A) (B) (C) (D)	65. (A) (B) (C) (D)
6. (A) (B) (C) (D)	26. (A) (B) (C) (D)	46. (A) (B) (C) (D)	66. (A) (B) (C) (D)
7. (A) (B) (C) (D)	27. (A) (B) (C) (D)	47. (A) (B) (C) (D)	67. (A) (B) (C) (D)
8. (A) (B) (C) (D)	28. (A) (B) (C) (D)	48. (A) (B) (C) (D)	68. (A) (B) (C) (D)
9. (A) (B) (C) (D)	29. (A) (B) (C) (D)	49. (A) (B) (C) (D)	69. (A) (B) (C) (D)
10. (A) (B) (C) (D)	30. (A) (B) (C) (D)	50. (A) (B) (C) (D)	70. (A) (B) (C) (D)
11. (A) (B) (C) (D)	31. (A) (B) (C) (D)	51. (A) (B) (C) (D)	71. (A) (B) (C) (D)
12. (A) (B) (C) (D)	32. (A) (B) (C) (D)	52. (A) (B) (C) (D)	72. (A) (B) (C) (D)
13. (A) (B) (C) (D)	33. (A) (B) (C) (D)	53. (A) (B) (C) (D)	73. (A) (B) (C) (D)
14. (A) (B) (C) (D)	34. (A) (B) (C) (D)	54. (A) (B) (C) (D)	74. (A) (B) (C) (D)
15. (A) (B) (C) (D)	35. (A) (B) (C) (D)	55. (A) (B) (C) (D)	75. (A) (B) (C) (D)
16. (A) (B) (C) (D)	36. (A) (B) (C) (D)	56. (A) (B) (C) (D)	76. (A) (B) (C) (D)
17. (A) (B) (C) (D)	37. (A) (B) (C) (D)	57. (A) (B) (C) (D)	77. (A) (B) (C) (D)
18. (A) (B) (C) (D)	38. (A) (B) (C) (D)	58. (A) (B) (C) (D)	78. (A) (B) (C) (D)
19. (A) (B) (C) (D)	39. (A) (B) (C) (D)	59. (A) (B) (C) (D)	79. (A) (B) (C) (D)
20. (A) (B) (C) (D)	40. (A) (B) (C) (D)	60. (A) (B) (C) (D)	80. (A) (B) (C) (D)

Section I - Verbal Ability

Questions 1-4 refer to the following passage.

Passage 1 - The Respiratory System

The respiratory system's function is to allow oxygen exchange through all parts of the body. The anatomy or structure of the exchange system, and the uses of the exchanged gases, varies depending on the organism. In humans and other mammals, for example, the anatomical features of the respiratory system include airways, lungs, and the respiratory muscles. Molecules of oxygen and carbon dioxide are passively exchanged, by diffusion, between the gaseous external environment and the blood. This exchange process occurs in the alveolar region of the lungs.

Other animals, such as insects, have respiratory systems with very simple anatomical features, and in amphibians even the skin plays a vital role in gas exchange. Plants also have respiratory systems but the direction of gas exchange can be opposite to that of animals.

The respiratory system can also be divided into physiological, or functional, zones. These include the conducting zone (the region for gas transport from the outside atmosphere to just above the alveoli), the transitional zone, and the respiratory zone (the alveolar region where gas exchange occurs). [17]

1. What can we infer from the first paragraph in this passage?

    a. Human and mammal respiratory systems are the same.

    b. The lungs are an important part of the respiratory system.

    c. The respiratory system varies in different mammals.

    d. Oxygen and carbon dioxide are passive exchanged by the respiratory system.

2. What is the process by which molecules of oxygen and carbon dioxide are passively exchanged?

    a. Transfusion

    b. Affusion

    c. Diffusion

    d. Respiratory confusion

3. What organ plays an important role in gas exchange in amphibians?

    a. The skin

    b. The lungs

    c. The gills

    d. The mouth

4. What are the three physiological zones of the respiratory system?

    a. Conducting, transitional, respiratory zones

    b. Redacting, transitional, circulatory zones

    c. Conducting, circulatory, inhibiting zones

    d. Transitional, inhibiting, conducting zones

Questions 5-8 refer to the following passage.

ABC Electric Warranty

ABC Electric Company warrants that its products are free from defects in material and workmanship. Subject to the conditions and limitations set forth below, ABC Electric will, at its option, either repair or replace any part of its products that prove defective due to improper workmanship or materials.

This limited warranty does not cover any damage to the product from improper installation, accident, abuse, misuse, natural disaster, insufficient or excessive electrical supply, abnormal mechanical or environmental conditions, or any unauthorized disassembly, repair, or modification.

This limited warranty also does not apply to any product on which the original identification information has been altered, or removed, has not been handled or packaged correctly, or has been sold as second-hand.

This limited warranty covers only repair, replacement, refund or credit for defective ABC Electric products, as provided above.

5. I tried to repair my ABC Electric blender, but could not, so can I get it repaired under this warranty?

    a. Yes, the warranty still covers the blender.

    b. No, the warranty does not cover the blender.

    c. Uncertain. ABC Electric may or may not cover repairs under this warranty.

6. My ABC Electric fan is not working. Will ABC Electric provide a new one or repair this one?

    a. ABC Electric will repair my fan

    b. ABC Electric will replace my fan

    c. ABC Electric could either replace or repair my fan or I can request either a replacement or a repair.

7. My stove was damaged in a flood. Does this warranty cover my stove?

    a. Yes, it is covered.

    b. No, it is not covered.

    c. It may or may not be covered.

    d. ABC Electric will decide if it is covered.

8. Which of the following is an example of improper workmanship?

    a. Missing parts

    b. Defective parts

    c. Scratches on the front

    d. None of the above

Questions 9 – 12 refer to the following passage.

Passage 3 – Mythology

The main characters in myths are usually gods or supernatural heroes. As sacred stories, rulers and priests have traditionally endorsed their myths and as a result, myths have a close link with religion and politics. In the society where a myth originates, the natives believe the myth is a true account of the remote past. In fact, many societies have two categories of traditional narrative—(1) "true stories", or myths, and (2) "false stories", or fables.

Myths generally take place during a primordial age, when the world was still young, prior to achieving its current form. These stories explain how the world gained its current form and why the culture developed its customs, institutions, and taboos. Closely related to myth are legend and folktale. Myths, legends, and folktales are different types of traditional stories. Unlike myths, folktales can take place at any time and any place, and the natives do not usually consider them true or sacred. Legends, on the other hand, are similar to myths in that many people have traditionally considered them true. Legends take place in a more recent time, when the world was much as it is today. In addition, legends generally feature humans as their main characters, whereas myths have super-human characters. [18]

9. We can infer from this passage that

 a. Folktales took place in a time far past, before civilization covered the earth

 b. Humankind uses myth to explain how the world was created

 c. Myths revolve around gods or supernatural beings; the local community usually accepts these stories as not true

 d. The only difference between a myth and a legend is the time setting of the story

10. The main purpose of this passage is

 a. To distinguish between many types of traditional stories, and explain the background of some traditional story categories

 b. To determine whether myths and legends might be true accounts of history

 c. To show the importance of folktales how these traditional stories made life more bearable in harder times

 d. None of the Above

11. How are folktales different from myths?

 a. Folktales and myth are the same

 b. Folktales are not true and generally not sacred and take place anytime

 c. Myths are not true and generally not sacred and take place anytime

 d. Folktales explained the formation of the world and myths do not

12. How are legends and myth similar?

 a. Many people believe legends and myths are true, myths take place in modern day, and legends are about ordinary people

 b. Many people believe legends and myths are true, legends take place in modern day, and legends are about ordinary people

 c. Many people believe legends and myths are true, legends take place in modern day, and myths are about ordinary people

 d. Many people believe legends and myths are not true, legends take place in modern day, and legends are about ordinary people

Questions 13-18 refer to the following passage.

Passage 4 – Myths, Legend and Folklore

Cultural historians draw a distinction between myth, legend and folktale simply as a way to group traditional stories. However, in many cultures, drawing a sharp line between myths and legends is not that simple. Instead of dividing their traditional stories into myths, legends, and folktales, some cultures divide them into two categories. The first category roughly corresponds to folktales, and the second is one that combines myths and legends. Similarly, we can not always separate myths from folktales. One society might consider a story true, making it a myth. Another society may believe the story is fiction, which makes it a folktale. In fact, when a myth loses its status as part of a religious system, it often takes on traits more typical of folktales, with its formerly divine characters now appearing as human heroes, giants, or fairies. Myth, legend, and folktale are only a few of the categories of traditional stories. Other categories include anecdotes and some kinds of jokes. Traditional stories, in turn, are only one category within the much larger category of folklore, which also includes items such as gestures, costumes, and music. [18]

13. The main idea of this passage is that

a. Myths, fables, and folktales are not the same thing, and each describes a specific type of story.

b. Traditional stories can be categorized in different ways by different people.

c. Cultures use myths for religious purposes, and when this is no longer true, the people forget and discard these myths.

d. Myths can never become folk tales, because one is true, and the other is false.

14. The terms myth and legend are

a. Categories that are synonymous with true and false.

b. Categories that group traditional stories according to certain characteristics.

c. Interchangeable, because both terms mean a story that is passed down from generation to generation.

d. Meant to distinguish between a story that involves a hero and a cultural message and a story meant only to entertain.

15. Traditional story categories not only include myths and legends, but

a. Can also include gestures, since some cultures passed these down before the written and spoken word.

b. In addition, folklore refers to stories involving fables and fairy tales.

c. These story categories can also include folk music and traditional dress.

d. Traditional stories themselves are a part of the larger category of folklore, which may also include costumes, gestures, and music.

16. This passage shows that

a. There is a distinct difference between a myth and a legend, although both are folktales.

b. Myths are folktales, but folktales are not myths.

c. Myths, legends, and folktales play an important part in tradition and the past, and are a rich and colorful part of history.

d. Most cultures consider myths to be true.

Questions 17-19 refer to the following passage.

Passage 5 – Insects

Humans regard certain insects as pests and attempt to control them with insecticides and many other techniques. Some insects damage crops by feeding on sap, leaves or fruits, a few bite humans and livestock, alive and dead, to feed on blood and some are capable of transmitting diseases to humans, pets and live-stock. Many other insects are considered ecologically beneficial and a few provide direct economic benefit. Silkworms and bees, for example, have been domesticated for the production of silk and honey, respectively. [19]

17. How do humans control insects?

a. By training them

b. Using insecticides and other techniques

c. In many different ways

d. Humans do not control insects

18. Why do humans control insects?

a. Because they do not like them

b. Because they damage crops

c. Because they damage buildings

d. Because they damage the soil

19. How do insects damage crops?

a. By feeding on crops

b. By transmitting disease

c. By laying eggs on crops

d. None of the above

Questions 20-24 refer to the following passage.

Passage 6 – Trees I

Trees are an important part of the natural landscape because they prevent erosion and protect ecosystems in and under their branches. Trees also play an important role in producing oxygen and reducing carbon dioxide in the atmosphere, as well as moderating ground temperatures. Trees are important elements in landscaping and agriculture, both for their visual appeal and for their crops, such as apples, and other fruit. Wood from trees is a building material, and a primary energy source in many developing countries. Trees also play a role in many of the world's mythologies. [20]

20. What are two reasons trees are important in the natural landscape?

    a. They prevent erosion and produce oxygen.

    b. They produce fruit and are important elements in landscaping.

    c. Trees are not important in the natural landscape.

    d. Trees produce carbon dioxide and prevent erosion.

21. What kind of ecosystems do trees protect?

    a. Trees do not protect ecosystems.

    b. Weather sheltered ecosystems.

    c. Ecosystems around the base and under the branches.

    d. All of the above.

22. Which of the following is true?

    a. Trees provide a primary food source in the developing world.

    b. Trees provide a primary building material in the developing world.

    c. Trees provide a primary energy source in the developing world.

    d. Trees provide a primary oxygen source in the developing world.

23. Why are trees important for agriculture?

    a. Because of their crops

    b. Because they shelter ecosystems

    c. Because they are a source of energy

    d. Because of their visual appeal

24. What do trees do to the atmosphere?

    a. Trees produce carbon dioxide and reduce oxygen.

    b. Trees product oxygen and carbon dioxide.

    c. Trees reduce oxygen and carbon dioxide.

    d. Trees produce oxygen and reduce carbon dioxide.

Questions 25 - 28 refer to the following passage.

Passage 7 – Trees II

With an estimated 100,000 species, trees represent 25 percent of all living plant species. The majority of tree species grow in tropical regions of the world and many of these areas have not been surveyed by botanists, making species diversity poorly understood. The earliest trees were tree ferns and horsetails, which grew in forests in the Carboniferous period. Tree ferns still survive, but the only surviving horsetails are no longer in tree form. Later, in the Triassic period, conifers and ginkgos, appeared, followed by flowering plants after that in the Cretaceous period. [20]

25. Do botanists understand the number of tree species?

    a. Yes, botanists know exactly how many tree species exit.

    b. No, the species diversity is not well understood.

    c. Yes, botanists have a general idea.

    d. No, botanists have no idea.

26. Where do most trees species grow?

    a. Most tree species grow in tropical regions.

    b. There is no one area where most tree species grow.

    c. Tree species grow in 25% of the world.

    d. There are 100,000 tree species.

27. What tree(s) survived from the Carboniferous period?

    a. 25% of all trees

    b. Horsetails

    c. Conifers

    d. Tree Ferns

28. Choose the correct list below, ranked from oldest to youngest trees.

a.   Flowering plants, conifers and ginkgos, tree ferns and horsetails.

b.   Tree ferns and horsetails, conifers and ginkgos, flowering plants.

c.   Tree ferns and horsetails, flowering plants, conifers and ginkgos.

d.   Conifers and ginkgos, tree ferns and horsetails, flowering plants.

Questions 29 - 30 refer to the following passage.

Lowest Price Guarantee

Get it for less. Guaranteed!

ABC Electric will beat any advertised price by 10% of the difference.

1) If you find a lower advertised price, we will beat it by 10% of the difference.

2) If you find a lower advertised price within 30 days* of your purchase we will beat it by 10% of the difference.

3) If our own price is reduced within 30 days* of your purchase, bring in your receipt and we will refund the difference.

*14 days for computers, monitors, printers, laptops, tablets, cellular & wireless devices, home security products, projectors, camcorders, digital cameras, radar detectors, portable DVD players, DJ and pro-audio equipment, and air conditioners.

29. I bought a radar detector 15 days ago and saw an ad for the same model only cheaper. Can I get 10% of the difference refunded?

a.   Yes. Since it is less than 30 days, you can get 10% of the difference refunded.

b.   No. Since it is more than 14 days, you cannot get 10% of the difference re-funded.

c.   It depends on the cashier.

d.   Yes. You can get the difference refunded.

30. I bought a flat-screen TV for $500 10 days ago and found an advertisement for the same TV, at another store, on sale for $400. How much will ABC refund under this guarantee?

a. $100

b. $110

c. $10

d. $400

Questions 31-33 refer to the following passage.

Passage 9 - Insects

Insects have segmented bodies supported by an exoskeleton, a hard outer covering made mostly of chitin. The segments of the body are organized into three distinctive connected units, a head, a thorax, and an abdomen. The head supports a pair of antennae, a pair of compound eyes, and three sets of appendages that form the mouthparts.

The thorax has six segmented legs and, if present in the species, two or four wings. The abdomen consists of eleven segments, though in a few species these segments may be fused together or very small.

Overall, there are 24 segments. The abdomen also contains most of the digestive, respiratory, excretory and reproductive internal structures. There is considerable variation and many adaptations in the body parts of insects especially wings, legs, antenna and mouthparts. [19]

31. How many units do insects have?

   a. Insects are divided into 24 units

   b. Insects are divided into 3 units

   c. Insects are divided into segments not units

   d. It depends on the species

32. Which of the following is true?

   a. All insects have 2 wings

   b. All insects have 4 wings

   c. Some insects have 2 wings

   d. Some insects have 2 or 4 wings

33. What is true of insect's abdomen?

   a. It contains some of the organs

   b. It is too small for any organs

   c. It contains all of the organs

   d. None of the above

Questions 34-37 refer to the following passage.

Passage 10 - The Circulatory System

The circulatory system is an organ system that passes nutrients (such as amino acids and electrolytes), gases, hormones, and blood cells to and from cells in the body to help fight diseases and help stabilize body temperature and pH levels.

The circulatory system may be seen strictly as a blood distribution network, but some consider the circulatory system as composed of the cardiovascular system, which distributes blood, and the lymphatic system, which distributes lymph. While humans, as well as other vertebrates, have a closed cardiovascular system (meaning that the blood never leaves the network of arteries, veins and capillaries), some invertebrate groups have an open cardiovascular system. The most primitive animal phyla lack circulatory systems. The lymphatic system, on the other hand, is an open system.

Two types of fluids move through the circulatory system: blood and lymph. The blood, heart, and blood vessels form the cardiovascular system. The lymph, lymph nodes, and lymph vessels form the lymphatic system. The cardiovascular system and the lymphatic system collectively make up the circulatory system.

The main components of the human cardiovascular system are the heart and the blood vessels. It includes: the pulmonary circulation, a "loop" through the lungs where blood is oxygenated; and the systemic circulation, a "loop" through the rest of the body to provide oxygenated blood. An average adult contains five to six quarts (roughly 4.7 to 5.7 liters) of blood, which consists of plasma, red blood cells, white blood cells, and platelets. Also, the digestive system works with the circulatory system to provide the nutrients the system needs to keep the heart pumping. [21]

34. What can we infer from the first paragraph?

    a. An important purpose of the circulatory system is that of fighting diseases.

    b. The most important function of the circulatory system is to give the person energy.

    c. The least important function of the circulatory system is that of growing skin cells.

    d. The entire purpose of the circulatory system is not known.

35. Do humans have an open or closed circulatory system?

    a. Open

    b. Closed

    c. Usually open, though sometimes closed

    d. Usually closed, though sometimes open

36. In addition to blood, what two components form the cardiovascular system?

    a. The heart and the lungs

    b. The lungs and the veins

    c. The heart and the blood vessels

    d. The blood vessels and the nerves

37. Which system, along with the circulatory system, helps provide nutrients to keep the human heart pumping?

    a. The skeletal system

    b. The digestive system

    c. The immune system

    d. The nervous system

Questions 38-41 refer to the following passage.

Passage 11 - Blood

Blood is a specialized bodily fluid that delivers nutrients and oxygen to the body's cells and transports waste products away.

In vertebrates, blood consists of blood cells suspended in a liquid called blood plasma. Plasma, which comprises 55% of blood fluid, is mostly water (90% by volume), and contains dissolved proteins, glucose, mineral ions, hormones, carbon dioxide, platelets and the blood cells themselves.

Blood cells are mainly red blood cells (also called RBCs or erythrocytes) and white blood cells, including leukocytes and platelets. Red blood cells are the most abundant cells, and contain an iron-containing protein called hemoglobin that transports oxygen through the body.

The pumping action of the heart circulates blood around the body through blood vessels. In animals with lungs, arterial blood carries oxygen from inhaled air to the tissues of the body, and venous blood carries carbon dioxide, a waste product of metabolism produced by cells, from the tissues to the lungs to be exhaled. [22]

38. What can we infer from the first paragraph in this passage?

    a. Blood is responsible for transporting oxygen to the cells.

    b. Blood is only red when it reaches the outside of the body.

    c. Each person has about six pints of blood.

    d. Blood's true function was only learned in the last century.

39. What liquid are blood cells suspended?

a. Plasma

b. Water

c. Liquid nitrogen

d. A mixture consisting largely of human milk

40. Which of these is not contained in blood plasma?

a. Hormones

b. Mineral ions

c. Calcium

d. Glucose

41. Which body part exhales carbon dioxide after venous blood has carried it from body tissues?

a. The lungs

b. The skin cells

c. The bowels

d. The sweat glands

Verbal Ability Part II – Vocabulary

42. Choose the adjective that means shocking, terrible or wicked.

a. Pleasantries

b. Heinous

c. Shrewd

d. Provencal

43. Choose the noun that means a person or thing that tells or announces the coming of someone or something.

a. Harbinger

b. Evasion

c. Bleak

d. Craven

44. Choose a word that means the same as the underlined word.

He wasn't especially generous. All the servings were very judicious.

a. Abundant

b. Careful

c. Extravagant

d. Careless

45. Fill in the blank.

Because of the growing use of _____ as a fuel, corn production has greatly increased.

a. Alcohol

b. Ethanol

c. Natural gas

d. Oil

46. Fill in the blank.

In heavily industrialized areas, the pollution of the air causes many to develop _____ diseases.

    a. Respiratory

    b. Cardiac

    c. Alimentary

    d. Circulatory

47. Choose the best definition of inherent.

    a. To receive money in a will

    b. An essential part of

    c. To receive money from a will

    d. None of the above

48. Choose the best definition of vapid.

    a. adj. tasteless or bland

    b. v. To inflict, as a revenge or punishment

    c. v. to convert into gas

    d. v. to go up in smoke

49. Choose the best definition of waif.

    a. n. a sick and hungry child

    b. n. an orphan staying in a foster home

    c. n. homeless child or stray

    d. n. a type of French bread eaten with cheese

50. Choose the adjective that means similar or identical.

    a. Soluble

    b. Assembly

    c. Conclave

    d. Homologous

51. Choose a word with the same meaning as the underlined word.

We used that operating system 20 years ago, now it is <u>obsolete</u>.

    a. Functional

    b. Disused

    c. Obese

    d. None of the Above

52. Choose the word with the same meaning as the underlined word

His bad manners really <u>rankle</u> me.

    a. Annoy

    b. Obsolete

    c. Enliven

    d. None of the above

53. Fill in the blank.

Because hydroelectric power is a _____ source of energy, its use is excellent for the environment.

    a. Significant

    b. Disposable

    c. Renewable

    d. Reusable

54. Choose the best definition of torpid.

    a. Fast

    b. Rapid

    c. Sluggish

    d. Violent

55. Choose the best definition of gregarious.

    a. Sociable

    b. Introverted

    c. Large

    d. Solitary

56. Choose the best definition of mutation.

    a. v. To utter with a loud and vehement voice

    b. n. change or alteration

    c. n. An act or exercise of will

    d. v. To cause to be one

57. Choose the best definition of lithe.

    a. adj. small in size

    b. adj. Artificial

    c. adj. flexible or plaint

    d. adj. fake

58. Choose the best definition of resent.

    a. adj. To express displeasure or indignation

    b. v. To cause to be one

    c. adj. Clumsy

    d. adj. strong feelings of love

59. Choose the adjective that means irrelevant not having substance or matter.

    a. Immaterial

    b. Prohibition

    c. Prediction

    d. Brokerage

60. Choose the adjective that means perfect, no faults or errors.

    a. Impeccable

    b. Formidable

    c. Genteel

    d. Disputation

61. Choose the best definition of pudgy.

    a. v. to draw general inferences

    b. Adj. fat, plump and overweight

    c. n. permanence

    d. adj. spoilt or bad condition

62. Choose the best definition of alloy.

    a. To mix with something superior

    b. To mix

    c. To mix with something inferior

    d. To purify

63. Fill in the blank.

The process required the use of highly _____ liquids, so fire extinguishers were everywhere in the factory.

    a. Erratic

    b. Combustible

    c. Stable

    d. Neutral

64. Choose the best definition for the underlined word.

We don't want to hear the whole thing. Just the <u>salient</u> facts please.

    a. Irrelevant

    b. Erroneous

    c. Relevant

    d. Trivial

65. Choose the best definition for the underlined word.

I don't know why he is being so nice. I am sure he has an <u>ulterior</u> motive.

    a. Inferior

    b. Additional

    c. Simplistic

    d. Unfortunate

66. Choose the noun that means ruling council of a military government.

    a. Retribution

    b. Counsel

    c. Virago

    d. Junta

67. Choose a noun that means someone who takes more time than necessary.

    a. Manager

    b. Haggard

    c. Laggard

    d. Expound

68. Choose an adjective that means lacking enthusiasm, strength or energy.

    a. Hapless

    b. Languid

    c. Ubiquitous

    d. Promiscuous

69. Choose a word that means the same as the underlined word.

I still don't know exactly. That isn't <u>conclusive</u> evidence.

    a. Undeterred

    b. Unrelenting

    c. Unfortunate

    d. Definitive

70. Choose the best definition of mollify.

    a. To anger

    b. To modify

    c. To irritate

    d. To soothe

71. Choose the best definition of redundant.

    a. Backup

    b. Necessary repetition

    c. Unnecessary repetition

    d. No repetition

72. Choose the best definition of raucous.

    a. Adj. Pedantic; academic; for teaching

    b. Adj. contemptuous, scornful

    c. adj. Not essential under the circumstances

    d. adj. harsh or rough sounding

73. Choose the noun that means a person of influence, rank or distinction.

    a. Consummate

    b. Sinister

    c. Accolade

    d. Magnate

74. Choose the word that means the same as the underlined word.

The warehouse went bankrupt so all of the furniture has to be <u>sold.</u>

    a. Dissected

    b. Liquidated

    c. Destroyed

    d. Bought

75. Choose the word that means the same as the underlined word.

He sold the property when he didn't even own it. The whole thing was a <u>fraud</u>.

    a. Hoax

    b. Feign

    c. Defile

    d. Default

76. Choose the best definition of bicker.

    a. Chat

    b. Discuss

    c. Argue

    d. Debate

77. Choose a noun that means a lingering disease or ailment of the human body.

    a. Treatment

    b. Frontal

    c. Malady

    d. Assiduous

78. Choose the word that means the same as the underlined word.

Just because she is supervisor, doesn't mean we have to <u>cower</u> in front of her.

    a. Foible

    b. Grovel

    c. Humiliate

    d. Indispose

79. Choose the best definition of maverick.

    a. Antagonist

    b. Conformist

    c. Unconventional

    d. Conventional

80. Choose the adjective that means relating to a wedding or marriage.

    a. Nefarious

    b. Fluctuate

    c. Nuptial

    d. Flatulence

Section II – Math

1. It is known that $x^2 + 4x = 5$. Then x can be

    a. 0

    b. -5

    c. 1

    d. Either (b) or (c)

2. $(a + b)2 = 4ab$. What is necessarily correct?

    a. $a > b$

    b. $a < b$

    c. $a = b$

    d. None of the Above

3. The sum of the digits of a 2-digit number is 12. If we switch the digits, the number we get will be greater than the initial one by 36. Find the initial number.

    a. 39

    b. 48

    c. 57

    d. 75

4. In a class of 83 students, 72 are present. What percent of student is absent?

    a. 12

    b. 13

    c. 14

    d. 15

5. Kate's father is 32 years older than Kate is. In 5 years, he will be five times older. How old is Kate?

    a. 2

    b. 3

    c. 5

    d. 6

6. If Lynn can type a page in p minutes, what portion of the page can she do in 5 minutes?

    a. $5/p$

    b. $p - 5$

    c. $p + 5$

    d. $p/5$

7. Find the mean of these set of numbers – 2.5, 10.2, 4.5, 1.25, 7.05, 20.8

    a. 7.6

    b. 45.6

    c. 7

    d. 1.25

8. If Sally can paint a house in 4 hours, and John can paint the same house in 6 hours, how long will it take for both of them to paint the house together?

    a. 2 hours and 24 minutes

    b. 3 hours and 12 minutes

    c. 3 hours and 44 minutes

    d. 4 hours and 10 minutes

9. A bullet weighing 350g is shot towards a target at a velocity of 250m/s. Calculate the momentum of the bullet?

    a. 1.4 kg x m/s towards target

    b. 87.5 kg x m/s towards target

    c. 87500 kg x m/s towards target

    d. 8.75 kg x m/s towards target

10. Using the quadratic formula, solve the quadratic equation: $x^2 - 9x + 14 = 0$

    a. 2 and 7

    b. -2 and 7

    c. -7 and -2

    d. -7 and 2

11. Employees of a discount appliance store receive an additional 20% off the lowest price on any item. If an employee purchases a dishwasher during a 15% off sale, how much will he pay if the dishwasher originally cost $450?

    a. $280.90

    b. $287.00

    c. $292.50

    d. $306.00

12. The sale price of a car is $12,590, which is 20% off the original price. What is the original price?

    a. $14,310.40

    b. $14,990.90

    c. $15,108.00

    d. $15,737.50

13. A goat eats 214 kg. of hay in 60 days, while a cow eats the same amount in 15 days. How long will it take them to eat this hay together?

    a. 37.5

    b. 75

    c. 12

    d. 15

14. Express 125% as a decimal.

    a. .125

    b. 12.5

    c. 1.25

    d. 125

15. What are the prime factors of 125?

    a. 5 x 25

    b. 5 x 5 x 5

    d. All of the above

    d. None of the above

16. Solve for x: 30 is 40% of x

    a. 60

    b. 90

    c. 85

    d. 75

17. Which of these object has greater momentum, a 2kg truck moving east at 3.5m/s or a 4.3kg truck moving south at 1.5m/s?

    a. First truck at 7 kg x m/s moving east

    b. Second truck at 7.45 kg x m/s due south

    c. First truck at 6.45 kg x m/s due east

    d. Second truck at 7 kg x m/s due south

18. 12 ½% of x is equal to 50. Solve for x.

    a. 300

    b. 400

    c. 450

    d. 350

19. Express 24/56 as a reduced common fraction.

    a. 4/9

    b. 4/11

    c. 3/7

    d. 3/8

20. What are the prime factors of 132?

    a. 4 x 3 x 11

    b. 2 x 2 x 2 x 3 x 11

    c. 2 x 6 x 11

    d. 2 x 2 x 3 x 11

21. Express 87% as a decimal.

    a. .087

    b. 8.7

    c. .87

    d. 87

22. 60 is 75% of x. Solve for x.

    a. 80

    b. 90

    c. 75

    d. 70

23. Find the median of these set of test scores taken from a class of students – 90, 80, 77, 86, 50, 91, 73, 66, 69, 45, 43, 65, 75

    a. 13

    b. 73

    c. 9

    d. 706

24. 4.7 + .9 + .01 =

    a. 5.5

    b. 6.51

    c. 5.61

    d. 5.7

25. .87 - .48 =

    a. .39

    b. .49

    c. .41

    d. .37

26. The physician ordered 100 mg Ibuprofen/kg of body weight; on hand is 230 mg/tablet. The child weighs 50 lb. How many tablets will you give?

    a. 10 tablets

    b. 5 tablets

    c. 1 tablet

    d. 12 tablets

27. Find the mode from these numbers – 7,2,3,9,6,5,1,4,8

    a. 1

    b. 5

    c. 9

    d. None of the above

28. Simplify 4³

    a. 20

    b. 32

    c. 64

    d. 108

29. The physician ordered 5 mL of Capacitate; 15 mL/tsp is on hand. How many teaspoons will you give?

    a. 0.05 tsp

    b. 0.03 tsp

    c. 0.5 tsp

    d. 0.3 tsp

30. Using the quadratic formula, solve the quadratic equation: x - 31/x = 0

    a. $-\sqrt{13}$ and $\sqrt{13}$
    b. $-\sqrt{31}$ and $\sqrt{31}$
    c. $-\sqrt{31}$ and $2\sqrt{31}$
    d. $-\sqrt{3}$ and $\sqrt{3}$

31. The manager of a weaving factory estimates that if 10 machines run on 100% efficiency for 8 hours, they will produce 1450 meters of cloth. However, due to some technical problems, 4 machines run of 95% efficiency and the remaining 6 at 90% efficiency. How many meters of cloth can these machines will produce in 8 hours?

    a. 1334 meters

    b. 1310 meters

    c. 1300 meters

    d. 1285 meters

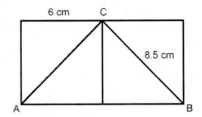

32. What is the perimeter of △ABC in the above shape?

    a. 25.5 cm

    b. 27 cm

    c. 30 cm

    d. 29 cm

33. Solve for x if, $10^2 \times 100^2 = 1000^x$

    a. x = 2

    b. x = 3

    c. x = -2

    d. x = 0

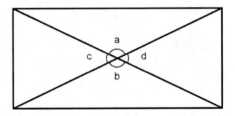

34. What is the sum of angles a, b, c and d in the rectangle above?

    a. 180°

    b. 360°

    c. 90°

    d. 120°

35. Find the mode from these test results – 2, 4, 2, 6, 4, 9, 6, 7, 2, 9, 7, 6, 4, 10, 10, 2, 6, 7, 9

     a. 2 and 9

     b. 2

     c. 2 and 6

     d. 2 and 7

36. Convert from scientific notation: 5.63×10^6

     a. 5,630,000

     b. 563,000

     c. 5630

     d. 0.000005.630

37. 30 mg is the same mass as:

     a. 0.0003 kg.

     b. 0.03 grams

     c. 300 decigrams

     d. 0.3 grams

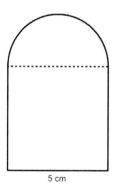

5 cm

38. What is the perimeter of the above shape?

     a. 17.5 π cm

     b. 20 π cm

     c. 15 π cm

     d. 25 π cm

39. 0.101 mm. =

     a. .0101 cm

     b. 1.01 cm

     c. 0.00101 cm

     d. 10.10 cm

40. Using the factoring method, solve the quadratic equation: $2x^2 - 3x = 0$

     a. 0 and 1.5

     b. 1.5 and 2

     c. 2 and 2.5

     d. 0 and 2

41. How much water can be stored in a cylindrical container 5 meters in diameter and 12 meters high?

     a. 223.65 ^{m3}

     b. 235.65 ^{m3}

     c. 240.65 ^{m3}

     d. 252.65 ^{m3}

42. Convert 0.045 to scientific notation.

     a. 4.5×10^{-2}

     b. 4.5×10^{2}

     c. 4.05×10^{-2}

     d. 4.5×10^{-3}

43. 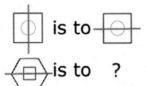 is to ⊡

is to ?

a. ⬡ b. ⬡

c. ⬦ d. ⬡

44. ◷ is to ◓

▥ is to ?

a. ▦ b. ▦

c. ▦ d. ▥

45. | is to ⬭

△ is to ?

a. ▷ b. ◁

c. ◇ d. △

46. 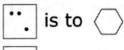 is to ⬡

⬚ is to ?

a. ⬠ b. ◯

c. ☐ d. △

47. Factor the polynomial $9x^2 - 6x + 12$.

    a. $3(x^2 - 2x + 9)$
    b. $3(3x^2 - 3x + 4)$
    c. $9(x^2 - 3x + 3)$
    d. $3(3x^2 - 2x + 4)$

48. 389 + 454 =

    a. 853
    b. 833
    c. 843
    d. 863

49. 9,177 + 7,204 =

    a. 16,4712
    b. 16,371
    c. 16,381
    d. 15,412

50. 2,199 + 5,832 =

    a. 8,331
    b. 8,041
    c. 8,141
    d. 8,031

Section III – Science

1. A soccer ball is kicked and travels at a velocity of 12 m/sec. After 60 seconds, it comes to a stop. What is the acceleration?

     a. -0.2 m/sec^2

     b. 0.2 m/sec^2

     c. 1 m/sec^2

     d. 0.5 m/sec^2

2. A molecule of water contains hydrogen and oxygen in a 1:8 ratio by mass. This is a statement of

     a. The law of multiple proportions

     b. The law of conservation of mass

     c. The law of conservation of energy

     d. The law of constant composition

3. Electrons play a critical role in

     a. Electricity

     b. Magnetism

     c. Thermal conductivity

     d. All of the above

4. An idea concerning a phenomena and possible explanations for that phenomena is a/an

     a. Theory.

     b. Experiment.

     c. Inference.

     d. Hypothesis.

5. Define chromosomes.

     a. Structures in a cell nucleus that carry genetic material.

     b. Consist of thousands of DNA strands.

     c. Total 46 in a normal human cell.

     d. All of the above

6. A base is

a. A compound that reacts with an acid to form a salt.

b. A molecule or ion that captures hydrogen ions.

c. A molecule or ion that donates an electron pair to form a chemical bond.

d. All of the above are true

7. Which disease of the circulatory system is one of the most frequent causes of death in North America?

a. The cold

b. Pneumonia

c. Arthritis

d. Heart disease

8. How fast can a person walk if they travel 1000 m in 20 minutes?

a. 25 meters

b. 50 meters

c. 100 meters

d. None of the above

9. A substance containing atoms of more than one element in a definite ratio is called a(n)

a. Compound.

b. Element.

c. Mixture.

d. Molecule.

10. Which of the following describes a plasma membrane?

a. Lipids with embedded proteins

b. An outer lipid layer and an inner lipid layer

c. Proteins embedded in lipid bilayer

d. Altering protein and lipid layers

11. Protein biosynthesis is defined as

a. The addition of protein to foods that lack it.

b. Ribosomes synthesizing proteins in the endoplasmic reticulum.

c. The process of proteasomes degrading cytoplasm.

d. Proteins "flowing" through the ER into the plasma membrane.

12. When we speak of separating organelles through centrifugation, we're speaking of

    a. Cell fractionation

    b. Flow cytometry

    c. Immunoprecipation

    d. Detergents

13. What is the difference between Strong Nuclear Force and Weak Nuclear Force?

a. The Strong Nuclear Force is an attractive force that binds protons and neutrons and maintains the structure of the nucleus, and the Weak Nuclear Force is responsible for the radioactive beta decay and other subatomic reactions.

b. The Strong Nuclear Force is responsible for the radioactive beta decay and other subatomic reactions, and the Weak Nuclear Force is an attractive force that binds protons and neutrons and maintains the structure of the nucleus.

c. The Weak Nuclear Force is feeble and the Strong Nuclear Force is robust.

d. The Strong Nuclear Force is a negative force that releases protons and neutrons and threatens the structure of the nucleus, and the Weak Nuclear Force is an attractive force that binds protons and neutrons and maintains the structure of the nucleus.

14. 1000 N force is applied to a concrete block that weights 500 pounds. How fast will this force accelerate the block?

    a. 1 m/sec^2

    b. 2 m/sec^2

    c. 3 m/sec^2

    d. 5 m/sec^2

15. What type of research deals with the quality, type or components of a group, substance, or mixture.

    a. Quantitative

    b. Dependent

    c. Scientific

    d. Qualitative

16. When a measurement is recorded, it includes the _____ _____, which are all the digits that are certain plus one uncertain digit.

    a. Major figures

    b. Significant figures

    c. Relative figures

    d. Relevant figures

17. The equation E = mc² is based on the _____, and states that _____ equals _____ times the _____².

    a. The equation $E = mc^2$ is based on the 2nd Law of Thermodynamics, and states that Mass equals Energy times (the Velocity of light)².

    b. The equation $E = mc^2$ is based on the Law of Conservation of Mass and Energy, and states that Energy equals Mass times (the Velocity of light)².

    c. The equation $E = mc^2$ is based on the 1st Law of Thermodynamics, and states that Mass equals Energy times (the Velocity of sound)².

    d. The equation $E = mc^2$ is based on the Law of Conservation of Mass and Energy, and states that the Velocity of light equals Energy times (the Mass)².

18. Describe a pH indicator.

    a. A pH indicator measures hydrogen ions in a solution and show pH on a color scale.

    b. A pH indicator measures oxygen ions in a solution and show pH on a color scale.

    c. A pH indicator many different types of ions in a solution and shows pH on a color scale

    d. None of the above

19. All acids turn blue litmus paper

    a. Blue

    b. Red

    c. Green

    d. White

20. What type of bonds involve a complete sharing of electrons and occurs most commonly between atoms that have partially filled outer shells or energy levels?

    a. Covalent

    b. Ionic

    c. Hydrogen

    d. Proportional

21. What can accept a hydrogen ion and can react with fats to form soaps?

    a. Acid

    b. Salt

    c. Base

    d. Foundation

22. Which, if any, of the following statements are true?

a. Water boils at approximately 100 °C (212 °F) at standard atmospheric pressure.

b. The boiling point is the temperature at which the vapor pressure is higher than the atmospheric pressure around the water.

c. Water boils at a higher temperature in areas of lower pressure.

d. All of the above statements are true.

23. Which gene, whose presence as a single copy, controls the expression of a trait?

a. Principal gene

b. Latent gene

c. Recessive gene

d. Dominant gene

24. What is the mathematical function that gives the amplitude of a wave as a function of position (and sometimes, as a function of time and/or electron spin)?

a. Wavelength

b. Frequency

c. Wavenumber

d. Wavefunction

25. Which of the following is not a habitat where bacteria commonly grow?

a. Soil

b. The vacuum of space

c. Radioactive waste

d. Deep in the earth's crust

26. Within taxonomy, plants and animals are considered two basic

a. Families

b. Kingdoms

c. Domains

d. Genus

27. How much force is needed to accelerate a car that weights 200 kg to 5 m/s²?

    a. 2000 N

    b. 4000 N

    c. 6000 N

    d. 8000 N

28. What is a chemical involved in, but not changed by, a chemical reaction by which chemical bonds are weakened and reactions accelerated.

    a. A propellant

    b. A reagent

    c. A catalyst

    d. None of the above

29. Organisms grouped into the _____ Kingdom include all unicellular organisms lacking a definite cellular arrangement such as _____ and _____ .

    a. Fungi, bacteria, algae

    b. Protista, bacteria, amphibian

    c. Protista, bacteria, algae

    d. Plantae, bacteria, algae

30. Which of these statements about metals are true?

    a. A metal is a substance that conducts heat and electricity.

    b. A metal is shiny and reflects many colors of light, and can be hammered into sheets or drawn into wire.

    c. All of these statements are true.

    d. About 80% of the known chemical elements are metals.

31. What type of bond does a reaction of elements with low electronegativity (almost empty outer shells) with elements with high electronegativity (mostly full outer shells) create?

    a. Hydrogen

    b. Covalent

    c. Ionic

    d. Nuclear

32. Which of the following is not an infectious bacterial disease?

   a. Cholera

   b. Anthrax

   c. Leprosy

   d. AIDS

33. Define a biological class.

   a. A collection of similar or like living entities.

   b. Two or more animals in a group, all having the same parent.

   c. All animals sharing the same living environment.

   d. All plant life that share the same physical properties.

34. Which, if any, of the following statements about prokaryotic cells is false?

   a. Prokaryotic cells include such organisms as E. coli and Streptococcus.

   b. Prokaryotic cells lack internal membranes and organelles.

   c. Prokaryotic cells break down food using cellular respiration and fermentation.

   d. All of these statements are true.

35. 1000 N force is applied to a concrete block that weights 500 pounds. How fast will this force accelerate the block?

   a. -2 m/sec^2

   b. 2 m/sec^2

   c. 4 m/sec^2

   d. 5 m/sec^2

36. What is the process of converting observed phenomena into data is called?

   a. Calculation

   b. Measurement

   c. Valuation

   d. Estimation

37. What law states that when two elements combine with each other to form more than one compound, the weights of one element that combine with a fixed weight of the other are in a ratio of small whole numbers?

    a. The Law of Multiple Proportions

    b. The Law of Definite Proportions

    c. The Law of the Conservation of Energy

    d. The Law of Averages

38. What word describes the wide diversity of sizes and shapes found in bacteria?

    a. Morphologies

    b. Cosmologies

    c. Proteins

    d. Spirilla

39. The mass number of an atom is

    a. The total number of particles that make it up.

    b. The total weight of an atom.

    c. The total mass of an atom.

    d. None of the above.

40. Which of these statements about mechanical energy is/are true?

    a. Mechanical energy is the energy that is possessed by an object due to its motion or due to its position.

    b. Mechanical energy can be either kinetic energy (energy of motion) or potential energy (stored energy of position).

    c. Objects have mechanical energy if they are in motion.

    d. All of the above.

41. What three processes are involved in cell division of Eukaryotic cells?

    a. Meiosis, mitosis, and interphase

    b. Meiosis, mitosis, and interphase

    c. Mitosis, kinematisis, and interphase

    d. Mitosis, cytokinesis, and interphase

42. The _____ _____ of an element equals the number of protons in an atomic nucleus, and, along with the element symbol is one of two alternate ways to label an element.

   a. Atomic unit

   b. Atomic number

   c. Atomic orbital

   d. Nuclear number

43. Which of the following statements, if any, are correct?

   a. pH is a measure of effective concentration of hydrogen ions in a solution, and is approximately related to the molarity of H+ by pH = - log [H+]

   b. pH is a measure of effective concentration of oxygen ions in a solution, and is approximately related to the molarity of O+ by pH = - log [O+]

   c. pH is a measure of effective concentration of hydrogen atoms in a solution, and is approximately related to the polarity of H+ by pH = - log [H+]

   d. Acidity is a measure of effective concentration of hydrogen ions in a solution, and is approximately related to the molarity of H+ by pH = - log [H+]

44. What chain of nucleotides plays an important role in the creation of new proteins?

   a. Deoxyribonucleic acid (DNA) is a chain of nucleotides that plays an important role in the creation of new proteins.

   b. Ribonucleic acid (RNA) is a chain of nucleotides that plays an important role in the creation of new proteins.

   c. There are no chains of nucleotides that play a role in the creation of proteins.

   d. None of the above.

45. How much force is needed to accelerate a car that weights 200 kg to 5 m/s²?

   a. 40 N

   b. 200 N

   c. 1000 N

   d. 1500 N

46. What law states that every chemical compound contains fixed and constant proportions (by weight) of its constituent elements?

   a. The Law of Multiple Proportions

   b. The Law of the Preservation of Matter

   c. The Law of the Conservation of Energy

   d. The Law of Definite Proportions

47. Four factors that affect rates of reaction are

a. Barometric pressure, particle size, concentration, and the presence of a facilitator.

b. Temperature, particle size, concentration, and the presence of a catalyst.

c. Temperature, container material, elevation, and the presence of instability.

d. Volatility, particle size, concentration, and the presence of a catalyst.

48. What is the term used for bacterial species which are spherical in shape?

a. Bacilli

b. Spirilla

c. Cocci

d. Spirochaetes

49. A practical test designed with the intention that its results will be relevant to a particular theory or set of theories is a/an _____.

a. Experiment

b. Practicum

c. Theory

d. Design

50. If 3 moles of sugar is dissolved to form 2 liters of a solution, calculate the molarity of the solution.

a. 1 M solution

b. 1.5 M solution

c. 2 M solution

d. 2.5 M solution

51. Electricity is a general term encompassing a variety of phenomena resulting from the presence and flow of electric charge. Which of the following statements about electricity is/are true?

a. Electrically charged matter is influenced by, and produces, electromagnetic fields.

b. Electric current is a movement or flow of electrically charged particles.

c. Electric potential is a fundamental interaction between the magnetic field and the presence and motion of an electric charge.

d. All of the statements are true.

52. Strong chemical bonds include

    a. Dipole - dipole interactions

    b. Hydrogen bonding

    c. Covalent or ionic bonds

    d. None of the above

53. A javelin is thrown into a field at 18 m/s. if the Javelin weighs 1.5 kg, what is the momentum?

    a. 1.2 kg x m/s into the field

    b. 12 kg x m/s into the field

    c. 27 kg x m/s into the field

    d. 2.7 kg x m/s into the field

54. Which of these object has greater momentum, a 2 kg truck moving east at 3.5 m/s or a 4.3 kg truck moving south at 1.5 m/s?

    a. The first truck at 7 kg x m/s moving east

    b. The second truck at 7.45 kg x m/s due south

    c. The first truck at 6.45 kg x m/s due east

    d. The second truck at 7 kg x m/s due south

55. What is the measure of an experiment's ability to yield the same or compatible results in different clinical experiments or statistical trials?

    a. Variability

    b. Validity

    c. Control measure

    d. Reliability

56. Genes control heredity in man and other organisms. This gene is

    a. a segment of RNA or DNA.

    b. a bead like structure on the chromosomes.

    c. a protein molecule.

    d. a segment of RNA.

57. One factor that affects rates of reaction is concentration. Which of these statements about concentration is/are correct?

    a. A higher concentration of reactants causes more effective collisions per unit time, leading to an increased reaction rate.

    b. A lower concentration of reactants causes more effective collisions per unit time, leading to an increased reaction rate.

    c. A higher concentration of reactants causes more effective collisions per unit time, leading to a decreased reaction rate.

    d. A higher concentration of reactants causes less effective collisions per unit time, leading to an increased reaction rate.

58. Describe each chemical element in the periodic table.

    a. Each chemical element has a unique atomic number representing the number of electrons in its nucleus.

    b. Each chemical element has a varying atomic number depending on the number of protons in its nucleus.

    c. Each chemical element has a unique atomic number representing the number of protons in its nucleus.

    d. None of the above.

59. Which of the following statements about nonmetals are true?

    a. A nonmetal is a substance that conducts heat and electricity poorly.

    b. The majority of the known chemical elements are nonmetals.

    c. A nonmetal is brittle or waxy or gaseous.

    d. All of the statements are true.

60. The molarity of 5 liters of a salt solution is 0.5 M of salt solution. Calculate the moles of salt in the solution.

    a. 2 Moles

    b. 2.5 Moles

    c. 2.75 Moles

    d. 3 Moles

61. A solution with a pH value of less than 7 is

    a. Acid solution

    b. Base solution

    c. Neutral pH solution

    d. None of the above

62. What is the distance between adjacent peaks (or adjacent troughs) on a wave?

a. Frequency

b. Wavenumber

c. Wave oscillation

d. Wavelength

63. An object that weighs 500 g is rolling along the road at 3.5 m/s. What is the momentum of the object?

a. 124.9 kg x m/s along road

b. 17. 50 kg x m/s along road

c. 1750 kg x m/s along road

d. 1.75 kg x m/s along road

64. Is a catalyst changed by a reaction?

a. Yes

b. No

c. It may be changed depending on the other chemicals

65. The _____ is the prediction that an observed difference is due to chance alone and not due to a systematic cause; this hypothesis is tested by statistical analysis, and either accepted or rejected.

a. Null hypothesis

b. Hypothesis

c. Control

d. Variable

66. In science, industry, and statistics, the _____ of a measurement system is the degree of closeness of measurements of a quantity to its actual (true) value.

a. Mistake

b. Uncertainty

c. Accuracy

d. Error

67. The horizontal rows of the periodic table are known as

    a. Groups

    b. Periods

    c. Series

    d. Columns

68. Which, if any, of these statements about solubility are correct?

    a. The solubility of a substance is its concentration in a saturated solution.

    b. Substances with solubilities much less than 1 g/100 mL of solvent are usually considered insoluble.

    c. A saturated solution is one which does not dissolve any more solute.

    d. All of these statements are correct.

69. Describe a valence shell.

    a. Is the shell corresponding to the highest value of principal quantum number in the atom.

    b. The valence electrons in this shell are on average closer to the nucleus than other electrons.

    c. They are rarely directly involved in chemical reaction.

    d. None of the above are true.

70. To calculate the Molarity of a solution when the solute is given in grams and the volume of the solution is given in milliliters, you must first

    a. Convert grams to moles, but leave the volume of solution in milliliters.

    b. Convert volume of solution in milliliters to liters, but leave grams to moles.

    c. Convert grams to moles, and convert volume of solution in milliliters to liters.

    d. None of the above.

71. What is the atomic number for Hydrogen?

    a. 11

    b. 2

    c. 1

    d. 5

72. The vertical columns of the periodic table are known as

   a. Series

   b. Groups

   c. Periods

   d. Columns

73. The ____ of a distribution is the difference between the maximum value and the minimum value.

   a. Distribution

   b. Range

   c. Mode

   d. Median

74. A cannon ball weighing 35 kg is shot from a cannon towards the east at 220m/s, calculate the momentum of the cannon ball.

   a. 7500 kg m/s east

   b. 7700 kg m/s east

   c. 8000 kg m/s east

   d. 8500 kg m/s east

75. Which, if any, of the following statements describing acids are correct?

   a. An acid is a compound containing detachable hydrogen ions.

   b. An acid is a compound that can accept a pair of electrons from a base.

   c. A and B are correct

   d. None of the above

Answer Key

1. B

We can infer an important part of the respiratory system are the lungs. From the passage, "Molecules of oxygen and carbon dioxide are passively exchanged, by diffusion, between the gaseous external environment and the blood. This exchange process occurs in the alveolar region of the lungs."

Therefore, one of the primary functions for the respiratory system is the exchange of oxygen and carbon dioxide, and this process occurs in the lungs. We can therefore infer that the lungs are an important part of the respiratory system.

2. C

The process by which molecules of oxygen and carbon dioxide are passively exchanged is diffusion.

This is a definition type question. Scan the passage for references to "oxygen," "carbon dioxide," or "exchanged."

3. A

The organ that plays an important role in gas exchange in amphibians is the skin.

Scan the passage for references to "amphibians," and find the answer.

4. A

The three physiological zones of the respiratory system are Conducting, transitional, respiratory zones.

5. B

This warranty does not cover a product that you have tried to fix yourself. From paragraph two, "This limited warranty does not cover ... any unauthorized disassembly, repair, or modification. "

6. C

ABC Electric could either replace or repair the fan, provided the other conditions are met. ABC Electric has the option to repair or replace.

7. B

The warranty does not cover a stove damaged in a flood. From the passage, "This limited warranty does not cover any damage to the product from improper installation, accident, abuse, misuse, natural disaster, insufficient or excessive electrical supply, abnormal mechanical or environmental conditions."

A flood is an "abnormal environmental condition," and a natural disaster, so it is not covered.

8. A

A missing part is an example of defective workmanship. This is an error made in the manufacturing process. A defective part is not considered workmanship.

9. B

The first paragraph tells us that myths are a true account of the remote past.

The second paragraph tells us that, "myths generally take place during a primordial age, when the world was still young, prior to achieving its current form."

Putting these two together, we can infer that humankind used myth to explain how the world was created.

10. A

This passage is about different types of stories. First, the passage explains myths, and then compares other types of stories to myths.

11. B

From the passage, "Unlike myths, folktales can take place at any time and any place, and the natives do not usually consider them true or sacred."

12. B

This question gives options with choices

for the three different characteristics of myth and legend. The options are,

- True or not true

- Takes place in modern day

- About ordinary people

For this type of question, where two things are compared for different characteristics, you can easily eliminate wrong answers using only one of the choices. Take myths: myths are believed to be true, do not take place in modern day, and are not about ordinary people.

Make a list as follows,

True or not true - True

Takes place in modern day - No

About ordinary people - No

Now check the options quickly. Option A is wrong (myths do not take place in modern day). Option B looks good. Put a check beside it. Option C is incorrect (myths are about ordinary people), and Option D is incorrect (myths are not true), so the answer must be Option B.

13. B
This passage describes the different categories for traditional stories. The other options are facts from the passage, not the main idea of the passage. The main idea of a passage will always be the most general statement. For example, Option A, Myths, fables, and folktales are not the same thing, and each describes a specific type of story. This is a true statement from the passage, but not the main idea of the passage, since the passage also talks about how some cultures may classify a story as a myth and others as a folktale.

The statement, from Option B, Traditional stories can be categorized in different ways by different people, is a more general statement that describes the passage.

14. B
Option B is the best choice, categories that group traditional stories according to certain characteristics.

Options A and C are false and can be eliminated right away. Option D is designed to confuse. Option D may be true, but it is not mentioned in the passage.

15. D
The best answer is D, traditional stories themselves are a part of the larger category of folklore, which may also include costumes, gestures, and music.

All of the other options are false. Traditional stories are part of the larger category of Folklore, which includes other things, not the other way around.

16. A
There is a distinct difference between a myth and a legend, although both are folktales.

17. B
The techniques for controlling insects are taken directly from the first sentence.

18. B
The inference is humans control pests because they damage crops.

19. A
Feeding on crops is the best choice, even though A and C are also correct.

20. A
Choice A is a re-wording of text from the passage.

21. C
This is taken directly from the passage.

22. C
Although trees are used as a building material, this is not their primary use. Trees are a primary energy source.

23. A
This is taken directly from the passage.

24. D
This question is designed to confuse by presenting different options for the two chemicals, oxygen and carbon dioxide. One is produced, and one is reduced. Read the passage carefully to see which is reduced and which is produced.

25. B
The inference is botanists have not surveyed all of the tropical areas so they do not know the number of species.

26. A
This is taken directly from the passage.

27. D
Tree-ferns survived the Carboniferous period. This is a fact-based question about the Carboniferous period. "Carboniferous" is an unusual word, so the fastest way to answer this question is to scan the passage for the word "Carboniferous" and find the answer.

28. B
Here is the passage with the oldest to youngest trees.

The earliest trees were [1] tree ferns and horsetails, which grew in forests in the Carboniferous period. Tree ferns still survive, but the only surviving horsetails are no longer in tree form. Later, in the Triassic period, [2] conifers and ginkgos, appeared, [3] followed by flowering plants after that in the Cretaceous period.

29. B
The time limit for radar detectors is 14 days. Since you made the purchase 15 days ago, you do not qualify for the guarantee.

30. B
Since you made the purchase 10 days ago, you are covered by the guarantee. Since it is an advertised price at a different store,

ABC Electric will "beat" the price by 10% of the difference, which is,

500 – 400 = 100 – difference in price

100 X 10% = $10 – 10% of the difference

The advertised lower price is $400. ABC will beat this price by 10% so they will refund $100 + 10 = $110.

31. B
From the first paragraph, "The segments of the body are organized into three distinctive connected units, a head, a thorax, and an abdomen."

This question tries to confuse 'segments' and 'units.'

32. D
This question tries to confuse. Read the passage carefully to find reference to the number of wings. "...if present in the species, two or four wings."

From this, we can conclude some insects have no wings, (if present ...) some have 2 wings and some have 4 wings.

33. A
The question asks about the abdomen and choices refer to organs in the abdomen. The passage says, "The abdomen also contains most of the digestive, respiratory, ... "

The choices are,

    a. It contains some of the organs.

    b. It is too small for any organs.

    c. It contains all of the organs.

    d. None of the above.

Choice A is true, but we need to see if there is better choice before answering. Choice B is not true. Choice C is not true since the relevant sentence says 'most' not 'all.' Choice D can be eliminated since

Choice A is true.

Given there is not better choice, Choice A is the best choice answer.

34. A
We can infer that an important purpose of the circulatory system is that of fighting diseases.

35. B
Humans have a closed circulatory system.

36. C
In addition to blood, the heart and the blood vessels form the cardiovascular system.

37. B
The digestive system, along with the circulatory system, helps provide nutrients to keep the human heart pumping.

38. A
We can infer that blood is responsible for transporting oxygen to the cells.

39. A
Human blood cells suspended in plasma.

40. C
Calcium is not contained in blood plasma.

From the passage, "[Blood Plasma] contains dissolved proteins, glucose, mineral ions, hormones, carbon dioxide, platelets and the blood cells themselves."

41. A
The lungs exhale the carbon dioxide after venous blood has been carried from body tissues.

42. B
Heinous: adj. shocking, terrible or wicked.

43. A
Harbinger: n. a person of thing that tells or announces the coming of someone or something

44. B
Judicious: Having, or characterized by, good judgment or sound thinking.

45. B
Ethanol: n. a colorless volatile flammable liquid C2H6O.

46. A
Respiratory: adj. Of, relating to, or affecting respiration or the organs of respiration.

47. B
Inherent: Naturally a part or consequence of something.

48. A
Vapid: adj. tasteless or bland.

49. C
Waif: n. homeless child or stray.

50. D
Homologous: adj. similar or identical.

51. B
Obsolete: adj. no longer in use; gone into disuse; disused or neglected.

52. A
Rankle: v. To cause irritation or deep bitterness.

53. D
Reusable

54. C
Torpid: adj. Lazy, lethargic or apathetic.

55. A
Gregarious: adj. Describing one who enjoys being in crowds and socializing.

56. B
Mutation: n. a change or alteration.

57. C
Lithe: adj. flexible or pliant.

58. A
Resent: v. to express displeasure or indignation.

59. A
Immaterial: adj. irrelevant not having substance or matter.

60. A
Impeccable: adj. perfect, no faults or errors.

61. B
Pudgy: adj. fat, plump or overweight.

62. C
Alloy: v. Mix or combine; often used of metals.

63. B
Combustible: adj. Able to catch fire and burn easily.

64. C
Salient: adj. Worthy of note; pertinent or relevant.

65. B
Ulterior: adj. beyond what is obvious or evident.

66. D
Junta: n. ruling council of a military government.

67. C
Laggard: n. someone who takes more time than necessary.

68. B
Languid: adj. lacking enthusiasm, strength or energy.

69. D
Conclusive: adj. Providing an end to something; decisive.

70. D
Mollify: v. To ease a burden; make less painful; to comfort.

71. C
Redundant: adj. Unnecessary repetition.

72. D
Raucous: adj. harsh or rough sounding.

73. D
Magnate: n. a person of influence, rank or distinction.

74. B
Liquidate: v. to convert assets into cash.

75. A
Hoax: n. To deceive (someone) by making them believe something which has been maliciously or mischievously fabricated.

76. C
Bicker: n. To quarrel in a tiresome, insulting manner.

77. C
Malady: n. A disease or ailment.

78. B
Grovel: To abase oneself before another person.

79. C
Maverick: n. Showing independence in thoughts or actions. Unconventional.

80. C
Nuptial: adj. Of or pertaining to wedding and marriage.

Section II – Math

1. D
$x^2 + 4x = 5$, $x^2 + 4x - 5 = 0$, $x^2 + 5x - x - 5 = 0$, factoring $x(x + 5) - 1(x + 5) = 0$, $(x + 5)(x-1)=0$. $x + 5 = 0$ or $x - 1 = 0$, $x = 0 - 5$ or $x = 0 + 1$, $x = -5$ or $x = 1$, either b or c.

2. C
Open parenthesis: $2a + 2b = 4ab$, divide both sides by 2 = $a + b = 2ab$ or $a + b = ab + ab$, therefore $a = ab$ and $b = ab$, therefore $a = b$.

3. B
Let the XY represent the initial number, $X + Y = 12$, $YX = XY + 36$, Only b = 48 satisfies both equations above from the given options.

4. B
Absent students = $83 - 72 = 11$. Percent of the absent students = $11/83 \times 100 = 13.25$ Reducing to two significant digits it will be 13.

5. B
Let the father's age=Y, and Kate's age=X, therefore Y=32+X, in 5yrs y=5x, substituting for Y will be 5x = 32+X, $5x - x = 32$, $4X=32$, $X= 32/8$, $x = 8$, Kate will be 8 in 5 yrs time, so Kate's present age = 8 - 5 = 3.

6. D
If Lynn can type a page in p minutes, then the portion of the page can she do in 5 minutes is p/5.

7. A
First add all the numbers $2.5 + 9.5 + 4.5 + 1.25 + 7.05 + 20.8 = 45.6$. Then divide by 6 (the number of data provided) = $45.6/6 = 7.6$

8. A
Let X represent the house, Sally paints X in 4hrs or ¼ X per 1hr or 60 minutes,

John paints X in 6 hours or at 1/6X per 1hr or 60mins. Working together, they will paint 1/4x + 1/6x in 1hr or 60minutes = 10/24x = 5/12x every 60 minutes, to paint x = 60 minutes x 12/5 = 144 minutes or 2 hrs and 24 minutes.

9. B
First convert 350g to kg = 350/1000 = 0.35kg. Momentum of bullet = 0.35 x 250 = 87.5 kg x m/s towards target

10. A
2 and 7

$$x^2 - 9x + 14 = 0$$

$$x_{1,2} = \frac{-(-9) \pm \sqrt{(-9)^2 - 4 \cdot 14}}{2 \cdot 1}$$

$$x_{1,2} = \frac{9 \pm \sqrt{81 - 56}}{2}$$

$$x_{1,2} = \frac{9 \pm \sqrt{25}}{2}$$

$$x_{1,2} = \frac{9 \pm 5}{2}$$

$$x_1 = \frac{9 + 5}{2} = 7$$

$$x_2 = \frac{9 - 5}{2} = 2$$

11. D
The cost of the dishwasher = $450, 15% discount = 15/100 x 450 = $67.5,
The new price = 450 – 67.5 = $382.5, 20% discount on lowest price = 20/100 x 382.5 = $76.5, so the final price = $306.

12. D
Original price = x,
80/100 = 12590/X,
80X = 1259000,
X = 15737.50.

13. C
Total hay = 214 kg,
The goat eats at a rate of 214/60 days = 3.6 kg per day.
The Cow eats at a rate of 214/15 = 14.3 kg per day,
Together they eat 3.6 + 14.3 = 17.9 per

day.

At a rate of 17.9 kg per day, they will consume 214 kg in 214/17.9 = 11.96 or 12 days approximately.

14. C

125/100 = 1.25

15 B

The smallest prime number that can divide 125 is 5. 125/5 = 25. 25/5 =5. Prime factors of 125 = 5 x 5 x5

16. D

40/100 = 30/X = 40X = 30 * 100 = 3000/40 = 75

17. A

Momentum of first object = 2 x 3.5 = 7; momentum of second truck = 4.3 x 1.5 = 6.45. First truck has more momentum at 7 kg x m/s moving east

18. B

12.5/100 = 50/X = 12.5X = 50 * 100 = 5000/12.5 = 400

19. C

24/56 = 3/7 (divide numerator and denominator by 8)

20. D

The smallest prime number to divide 132 is 2. 132/2 = 66. 66/2 = 33. 33/3 = 11. 11 cannot be divided further by a prime number other than 11. The prime numbers of 132 = 2 x 2 x 3 x 11

21. C

Converting percent to decimal – divide percent by 100 and remove the % sign. 87% = 87/100 = .87

22. A

60 has the same relation to X as 75 to 100 – so

60/X = 75/100

6000 = 75X

X = 80

23. B

First arrange the numbers in a numerical sequence – 43, 45, 50, 65, 66, 69, 73, 75, 77, 80, 86, 90, 91. Next find the middle number. The median = 73

24. C

4.7 + .9 + .01 = 5.61

25. A

.87 - .48 = .39

26. A

Step 1: Set up the formula to calculate the dose to be given in mg as per weight of the child:-

Dose ordered X Weight in Kg = Dose to be given

Step 2: 100 mg X 23 kg = 2300 mg

(Convert 50 lb to Kg, 1 lb = 0.4536 kg, hence 50 lb = 50 X 0.4536 = 22.68 kg approx. 23 kg)

2300 mg/230 mg X 1 tablet/1 = 2300/230 = 10 tablets

27. D

Simply find the most recurring number. All the numbers in the series appeared only once. The answer is No Mode

28. C

4 x 4 x 4 = 64

29. D

5 ml/15 ml kX 1 tsp/1 = 5/15 = 0.3 tsp

30. B

$-\sqrt{31}$ and $\sqrt{31}$

$$x - \frac{31}{x} = 0$$

$$\frac{x^2 - 31}{x} = 0 \Rightarrow x^2 - 31 = 0$$

$$x_{1,2} = \frac{0 \pm \sqrt{-4 \cdot (-31)}}{2}$$

$$x_{1,2} = \frac{\pm 2\sqrt{31}}{2}$$

$$x_{1,2} = \pm\sqrt{31}$$

$$x_1 = \sqrt{31}$$

$$x_2 = -\sqrt{31}$$

31. A
At 100% efficiency 1 machine produces 1450/10 = 145 m of cloth.
At 95% efficiency, 4 machines produce 4 X 0.95 X 145 = 551 m of cloth.
At 90% efficiency, 6 machines produce 6 X 0.90 X 145 = 783 m of cloth.

Total cloth produced = 551 + 783 = 1334 m

32. D
Perimeter of triangle ABC within two squares.
Perimeter = sum of the sides.
Perimeter = 8.5 + 8.5 + 6 + 6
Perimeter = 29 cm.

33. A
10 x 10 x 100 x 100 = 1000^x, =100 x 10,000 = 1000^x, = 1,000,000 = 1000^x = x =2

34. B
a + b + c + d = ?
The sum of angles around a point is 360°
a + b + c + d = 360°

35. C
Simply find the most recurring number.
The most occurring numbers in the series is 2 and 6

36. A
The scientific notation is in the positive so we shift the decimal 6 places to the right. Thus it is 5,630,000

37. D
There are 1000 mg in a gram. 30/1000 = 0.03 grams. To divide by 1000, move the decimal 3 places to the left. =

38. A
The shape is made of a square and a semi circle. Calculate the perimeter of each and add.
Perimeter = 3 sides of the square + ½ circumference of the circle.

= (3 x 5) + ½(5 π)
= 15 + 2.5 π
Perimeter = 17.5 π cm

39. A
There are 10 mm in a cm. 0.101/10 = .0101. To divide by 10, move the decimal 1 place to the left.

40. A
0 and 1.5
$2x^2 - 3x = 0$
x(2x - 3)
x = 0 or 2x - 3 =0
x = 0 or x = 3/2
x = 0 or x = 1.5

41. B
The formula for the volume of cylinder is = π r^2h
Where π is 3.142, r is radius of the cross sectional area, and h is the height.
So the volume will be = 3.142 × 2.5^2 × 12 = 235.65m^3.

42. A
The decimal point moves 2 spaces to the left to be placed after 4, which is the first non-zero number. 4.5 x 10^{-2} The exponent is negation since the decimal moved left.

43. D
The relation is the same figure rotated.

44. D
The shaded area is divided in half in the second figure.

45. D
The relation is the same figure rotated to the right.

46. B
The relation is the number of dots is one-half the number of sides.

47. D

$3(3x^2 - 2x + 4)$

$9x^2 - 6x + 12 = 3 * 3x^2 - 2 * 3x + 3 * 4 =$

$3(3x^2 - 2x + 4)$

48. C

$389 + 454 = 843$

49. C

$9,177 + 7,204 = 16,381$

50. D

$2,199 + 5,832 = 8,031$

Section V – Science

1. A

The formula for acceleration = $A = (V_f - V_0)/t$

so $A = (0 - 12)/60$ sec $= -0.2$ m/sec^2

2. A

The Law of Multiple Proportions states that when two elements combine with each other to form more than one compound, the weights of one element that combine with a fixed weight of the other are in a ratio of small whole numbers.

3. D

All of the above are true. Electrons play an essential role in electricity, magnetism, and thermal conductivity.

4. D

An idea concerning a phenomena and possible explanations for that phenomena is an hypothesis.

5. D

All of the above. Chromosomes are

　　a. Structures in a cell nucleus that carry genetic material.

　　b. Consist of thousands of DNA strands.

　　c. Total 46 in a normal human cell.

6. D

All of the statements about bases are true.

　　a. A compound that reacts with an acid to form a salt.

　　b. A molecule or ion that captures hydrogen ions.

　　c. A molecule or ion that donates an electron pair to form a chemical bond.

7. D

The circulatory system disease that is one of the most frequent causes of death in North America is heart disease.

8. B

Speed = (total distance traveled)/(total time taken)

X = 1000m/20 minutes

X = 50 meters

9. A

A chemical compound is a chemical substance comprising atoms from two or more elements in a specific ration as expressed in the chemical formula i.e., H2O

10. C

The plasma membrane or cell membrane protects the cell from outside forces. It consists of the lipid bilayer with embedded proteins

11. C

Protein biosynthesis is defines as, ribosomes synthesizing proteins in the endoplasmic reticulum. This process, also known as protein biosynthesis, is a process within the cell by which the substrates convert to products of higher complexity.

12. A

Cell fractionation. Fractionation is important because it purifies the cell and its parts.

13. A

The Strong Nuclear Force is an attractive force that binds protons and neutrons and maintains the structure of the nucleus, and the Weak Nuclear Force is responsible for the radioactive beta decay and other subatomic reactions.

14. B
Force = Mass times Acceleration Measured in Newtons.
1000 = 500 x A
A = 1000/500 = 2 m/s^2

15. D
Qualitative research deals with the quality, type or components of a group, substance, or mixture.

16. B
The equation E = mc^2 is based on the Law of Conservation of Mass and Energy, and states that Energy equals Mass times the Velocity of light^2.

17. B
When a measurement is recorded, it includes the significant figures, which are all the digits that are certain plus one uncertain digit.

18. A
A pH indicator measures hydrogen ions in a solution and show pH on a color scale.

19. B
Acids turns blue litmus paper red, base turns red litmus paper blue.

20. A
Covalent bonds involve a complete sharing of electrons and occurs most commonly between atoms that have partially filled outer shells or energy levels.

21. C
A base is any substance that can accept a hydrogen ion and can react with fats to form soaps.

22. A
Water boils at approximately 100 °C (212 °F) at standard atmospheric pressure.

23. D
The dominant gene controls the expression of a trait.

24. D
Wavefunction is a mathematical function that gives the amplitude of a wave as a function of position (and sometimes, as a function of time and/or electron spin).

Note: Wavefunctions are used in chemistry to represent the behavior of electrons bound in atoms or molecules.

25. B
The vacuum of space is an environment where bacteria do not commonly exit. The nature of outer space, including intense cold and lack of oxygen, makes it difficult for even most bacteria to grow.

26. B
Plants and animals are kingdoms. There are six recognized kingdoms: Animalia, Plantae, Protista, Fungi, Bacteria, and Archaea.

27. C
Force = Mass times Acceleration Measured in Newtons.
F = 2000 kg X 3 m/sec^2 = 6000 N

28. C
A catalyst is a chemical involved in, but not changed by, a chemical reaction by which chemical bonds are weakened and reactions accelerated.

29. C
Organisms grouped into the **Protista** Kingdom include all unicellular organisms lacking a definite cellular arrangement such as **bacteria** and **algae.**

30. C
All of these statements are true.

A metal is a substance that conducts

heat and electricity.

A metal is shiny and reflects many colors of light, and can be hammered into sheets or drawn into wire.

About 80% of the known chemical elements are metals.

31. C
The reaction of elements with low electronegativity(almost empty outer shells) with elements with high electronegativity (mostly full outer shells) gives rise to Ionic bonds.

32. D
AIDS (or Acquired Immune Deficiency Syndrome) is carried by a virus, not bacteria.

33. A
A collection of similar or like living entities. Class has the same meaning in biology as rank. Common classes or ranks include species, order, and phylum.

34. D
All of these statements are true.

> a. Prokaryotic cells include such organisms as E. coli and Streptococcus.
>
> b. Prokaryotic cells lack internal membranes and organelles.
>
> c. Prokaryotic cells break down food using cellular respiration and fermentation.

35. B
Force = Mass times Acceleration Measured in Newtons.
1000 = 500 x A
A = 1000/500 = 2 m/s²

36. B
The process of converting observed phenomena into data is called measurement.

37. A
The Law of Multiple Proportions states that when two elements combine with each other to form more than one compound, the weights of one element that combine with a fixed weight of the other are in a ratio of small whole numbers.

38. A
Morphology is defined as the field that studies the relationship between structures in living organisms.

39. A
The mass number of an atom is the total number of particles (protons and neutrons) that make it up.

40. A
All of the statements are true.

> a. Mechanical energy is the energy that is possessed by an object due to its motion or due to its position.
>
> b. Mechanical energy can be either kinetic energy (energy of motion) or potential energy (stored energy of position).
>
> c. Objects have mechanical energy if they are in motion

41. D
In Eukaryotic cells, the cell cycle is the cycle of events involving cell division, including mitosis, cytokinesis, and interphase.

42. B
The atomic number of an element equals the number of protons in an atomic nucleus, and, along with the element symbol is one of two alternate ways to label an element.

43. A
pH is a measure of effective concentration of hydrogen ions in a solution, and is approximately related to the molarity of H+ by pH = - log [H+]

44. B

Ribonucleic acid (RNA) is a chain of nucleotides that plays an important role in the creation of new proteins.

45. C

Force = Mass times Acceleration Measured in Newtons.
F = 200 X 5 = 1000 N

46. D

The Law of Definite Proportions states that every chemical compound contains fixed and constant proportions (by weight) of its constituent elements.

47. B

Four factors that affect rates of reaction are: Temperature, particle size, concentration, and the presence of a catalyst.

48. C

Spherical bacteria are Cocci. Along with bacilli, this is one of the two major structures for bacteria.

49. A

A practical test designed with the intention that its results will be relevant to a particular theory or set of theories is an experiment.

50. B

The formula for calculating molarity when the moles of the solute and liters of the solution are given is = moles of solute/ liters of solution.
Moles of Solute = 3 moles of sugar
Solution liters = 3 liters
Molarity of solution = ?

Therefore: molarity of the solution = 3 moles of solvent/ 2 liters of solution = 1.5 M solution.

51. D

All of the statements are true.

a. Electrically charged matter is influenced by, and produces, electromagnetic fields.

b. Electric current is a movement or flow of electrically charged particles.

c. Electric potential is a fundamental interaction between the magnetic field and the presence and motion of an electric charge.

52. C

Covalent or ionic bonds are considered "strong bonds."

53. C

P = 1.5 x 18 = 27 kg x m/s into the field.

54. A

Momentum of first object = 2 x 3.5 = 7; momentum of second truck = 4.3 x 1.5 = 6.45. First truck has more momentum at 7 kg x m/s moving east.

55. D

Reliability refers to the measure of an experiment's ability to yield the same or compatible results in different clinical experiments or statistical trials.

56. A

Genes are made from a long molecule called DNA, which is copied and inherited across generations. DNA is made of simple units that line up in a particular order within this large molecule. The order of these units carries genetic information, similar to how the order of letters on a page carries information. The language used by DNA is called the genetic code, which lets organisms read the information in the genes. This information is the instructions for constructing and operating a living organism.

57. A

A higher concentration of reactants causes more effective collisions per unit time, leading to an increased reaction rate.

58. C

Each chemical element has a unique atomic number representing the number of protons in its nucleus.

59. D
All of these statements are about non-metals are true.

> a. A nonmetal is a substance that conducts heat and electricity poorly.
>
> b. The majority of the known chemical elements are nonmetals.
>
> c. A nonmetal is brittle or waxy or gaseous.

60. B
Moles of solute = ? or X
Solutions liters = 5 liters
Molarity of solution = 0.5 M

Therefore: X moles/5 liters of solution = 0.5 or X/5 = 0.5
So X = 5/0.5
X = 2.5
Mole of salt in the solution is 2.5 moles

61. A
A solution with a pH value of less than 7 is acid. A pH value of 7 is neutral.

62. D
Wavelength is defined as the distance between adjacent peaks (or adjacent troughs) on a wave.

Note: Varying the wavelength of light changes its color; varying the wavelength of sound changes its pitch.

63. D
First convert 500 g to kg = 500/1000 = 0.5 kg, momentum = 0.5 x 3.5 = 1.75 kg x m/s along the road.

64. B
A catalyst is never changed in a chemical reaction.

65. A
The prediction that an observed difference is due to chance alone and not due to a systematic cause; this hypothesis is tested by statistical analysis, and accepted or rejected is the **null hypothesis**.

66. C
In science and engineering, the **accuracy** of a measurement system is the degree of closeness of measurements of a quantity to its actual (true) value.

67. B
The horizontal rows from right to left of the periodic table are known as periods and elements on a row share the same number of electron shells.

68. D
All of the statements about solubility are correct.

> a. The solubility of a substance is its concentration in a saturated solution.
>
> b. Substances with solubilities much less than 1 g/100 mL of solvent are usually considered insoluble.
>
> c. A saturated solution is one which does not dissolve any more solute.

69. A
A valence shell is the shell corresponding to the highest value of principal quantum number in the atom.

70. C
To calculate the Molarity of a solution when the solute is given in grams and the volume of the solution is given in milliliters, you must first **convert grams to moles, and convert volume of solution in milliliters to liters.**

71. C
Hydrogen is the first element listed on the periodic table. The atomic number for hydrogen is 1.

72. B

Vertical columns on the periodic table are called groups. There are 18 groups on the table. Elements on the same group each have the same number of electrons on their outermost shell.

73. B

The **range** of a distribution is the difference between the maximum value and the minimum value.

74. B

Formula - P= kg x m/s
= 35kg x 220 m/s
= 7700 kg x m/s east

75. C

A and B are correct.
An acid is a compound containing detachable hydrogen ions.
An acid is a compound that can accept a pair of electrons from a base.

Conclusion

CONGRATULATIONS! You have made it this far because you have applied yourself diligently to practicing for the exam and no doubt improved your potential score considerably! Getting into a good school is a huge step in a journey that might be challenging at times but will be many times more rewarding and fulfilling. That is why being prepared is so important.

Study then Practice and then Succeed!

Good Luck!

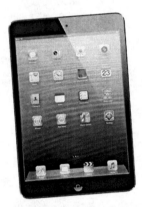

FREE Ebook Version

Download a FREE Ebook version of the publication!

Suitable for tablets, iPad, iPhone, or any smart phone.

Go to http://tinyurl.com/ne3t6nm

Register for Free Updates and More Practice Test Questions

Register your purchase at www.test-preparation.ca/register.html for fast and convenient access to updates, errata, free test tips and more practice test questions.

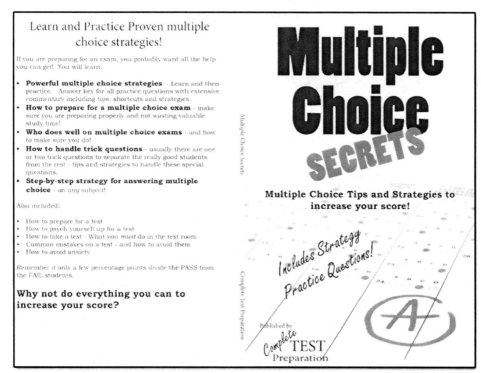

Multiple Choice Secrets!

Learn to increase your score using time-tested secrets for answering multiple choice questions!

This practice book has everything you need to know about answering multiple choice questions on a standardized test!

You will learn 12 strategies for answering multiple choice questions and then practice each strategy with over 45 reading comprehension multiple choice questions, with extensive commentary from exam experts!

Maybe you have read this kind of thing before, and maybe feel you don't need it, and you are not sure if you are going to buy this Book.

Remember though, it only a few percentage points divide the PASS from the FAIL students.

Even if our multiple choice strategies increase your score by a few percentage points, isn't that worth it?

Go to www.multiple-choice.ca start learning multiple choice secrets today!

Endnotes

Text where noted below is used under the Creative Commons Attribution-ShareAlike 3.0 License

http://en.wikipedia.org/wiki/Wikipedia:Text_of_Creative_Commons_Attribution-Share-Alike_3.0_Unported_License

1 Immune System. In *Wikipedia*. Retrieved November 12, 2010 from, http://en.wikipedia.org/wiki/Immune_system.

2 White Blood Cell. In *Wikipedia*. Retrieved November 12, 2010 from en.wikipedia.org/wiki/White_blood_cell.

3 Convection. In *Wikipedia*. Retrieved November 12, 2010 from en.wikipedia.org/wiki/Convection

4 Tight Junction. In *Wikipedia*. Retrieved November 12, 2010 from http://en.wikipedia.org/wiki/Tight_junction.

5 Biology. In *Wikipedia*. Retrieved May 10, 2012 from http://en.wikipedia.org/wiki/Biology.

6 Cell Structure. http://en.wikipedia.org/wiki/File:Animal_cell_structure_en.svg.

7 Phylum. In *Wikipedia*. Retrieved January 20, 2013 from http://en.wikipedia.org/wiki/Phylum

8 Chemistry. In *Wikipedia*. Retrieved May 10, 2012 from http://en.wikipedia.org/wiki/Chemistry.

9 Acceleration. In *Wikipedia*. Retrieved March 22, 2013 from http://en.wikipedia.org/wiki/Acceleration.

10 Infectious Disease. In *Wikipedia*. Retrieved November 12, 2010 from en.wikipedia.org/wiki/Infectious_disease.

11 Virus. In *Wikipedia*. Retrieved November 12, 2010 from en.wikipedia.org/wiki/Virus.

12 Cloud. In *Wikipedia*. Retrieved November 12, 2010 from http://en.wikipedia.org/wiki/Clouds.

13 Butterfly. In *Wikipedia*. Retrieved November 12, 2010 from en.wikipedia.org/wiki/Butterfly.

14 U.S. Navy Seal. In *Wikipedia*. Retrieved November 12, 2010 from en.wikipedia.org/wiki/United_States_Navy_SEALs.

15 Gardening. In *Wikipedia*. Retrieved January 2, 2012 from en.wikipedia.org/wiki/Gardening.

16 Coral Reef. In *Wikipedia*. Retrieved January 2, 2012 from http://en.wikipedia.org/wiki/Coral_reef.

17 Respiratory System. In *Wikipedia*. Retrieved November 12, 2010 from en.wikipedia.org/wiki/Respiratory_system.

18 Mythology. In *Wikipedia*. Retrieved November 12, 2010 from en.wikipedia.org/wiki/Mythology.

19 Insect. In *Wikipedia*. Retrieved November 12, 2010 from en.wikipedia.org/wiki/Insect.

20 Tree. In *Wikipedia*. Retrieved November 12, 2010 from en.wikipedia.org/wiki/Tree.

21 Circulatory System. In *Wikipedia*. Retrieved November 12, 2010 from en.wikipedia.org/wiki/Circulatory_system.

22 Blood. In *Wikipedia*. Retrieved November 12,2010 from http://en.wikipedia.org/wiki/Blood.

CPSIA information can be obtained at www.ICGtesting.com
Printed in the USA
LVOW09s0526130314

377224LV00004B/24/P

9 781927 358641